Contents

Nursing Older People

A Guide to Practice in Care Homes

Edited by Susan Carmody and Sue Forster
Revised for the UK by Nicky Hayes

Radcliffe Publishing
Oxford • San Francisco

Radcliffe Publishing Ltd
18 Marcham Road
Abingdon
Oxon OX14 1AA
United Kingdom

www.radcliffe-oxford.com
Electronic catalogue and worldwide online ordering.

This book was originally published in Melbourne, Australia by Ausmed Publications Pty Ltd

Palliative Care Nursing: A Guide to Practice
First edition published by Ausmed Publications Pty Ltd, 1999; reprinted 1999, 2001.
This second edition (completely revised and rewritten) first published by
Ausmed Publications Pty Ltd 2003.

British Library Cataloguing in Publication Data

A catalogue record for this book is available from the British Library

ISBN 1 85775 635 5

Typeset by Egan-Reid Ltd, Auckland, New Zealand
Printed and bound by T J International Ltd, Padstow, Cornwall, UK

Dedication

This book is dedicated to the memories of

Joyce Carmody
(mother of Susan Carmody)

and

James Forster
(father of Sue Forster)

Intelligent, dynamic, well-loved, and admired, they lived their lives to the full and had a wisdom and love of life that motivated others.

'But search the land of living men,
Where wilt thou find their like agen?'
WALTER SCOTT (1771–1832)
Scottish novelist, *Marmion*, 1

'To live in the hearts we leave behind,
Is not to die'
THOMAS CAMPBELL (1777–1844)
Hallowed Ground

'To die completely, a person must not only forget but be forgotten, and he who is not forgotten is not dead'
SAMUEL BUTLER (1835–1902)
English writer and satirist

Foreword

Pauline Ford

Nursing in Care Homes has become an increasingly important area and this book recognises the role of expert nursing in Care Homes. This is timely, as there is currently tremendous change and challenge in the provision of health and social care. The debate continues about the needs of older people living in Care Homes and the nursing contribution, with a particular focus on social care and a lack of recognition of the contributions that nursing can and does make to health and well being.

Crucially, this book sets out to address the nurse's contribution to the health and well being of older people living in Care Homes. It rightly focuses on a range of health needs that residents in Care Homes may present with. Nurses working with older people often express frustration that their role is under-recognised and under-valued. This book goes some way to help redress the balance by focusing on some of the areas where nurses have long demonstrated good practice. It can be seen as a celebration of all that is good in nursing. I believe that to practice nursing in a person-centred way is only possible if the nurse holds a value system that demonstrates a level of relating that truly values the 'other' in that relationship. Such an approach is implicit within this book and focuses on the human aspects of nursing. The challenge for us as nurses is how to maintain a person-centred approach whilst delivering specific health-related nursing interventions. This book will help nurses achieve this whilst working in a world of healthcare which is performance and fiscally driven. The need to hold on to the humanistic elements of care is central to best practice in nursing older people who live in Care Homes.

Pauline Ford
Advisor in Gerontological Nursing
Royal College of Nursing
June 2004

Preface

Susan Carmody and Sue Forster

Nursing older people is a specialised field of nursing. Although care of older people has been part of nursing since the beginning of the profession, it is only in more recent times that this specialty has 'come of age'. With increased life expectancy, the older population has grown markedly throughout the world. In parallel with this, a plethora of research means that nurses now have an ever-increasing database to guide their practice. No longer can effective nursing of older people rely on the ethical domain alone. Contemporary effective nursing for older people now requires sound scientific knowledge if care is to be provided on a rational basis. This does not mean that ethical issues are neglected. On the contrary, a greater emphasis on sound evidence-based nursing practice in care of older people means that nurses must incorporate their traditional ethical approach with sound modern scientific knowledge in an holistic model of care.

This book is written by clinicians for clinicians. Each chapter illustrates contemporary nursing practice pertinent to a specific area of care. The content of each chapter incorporates accepted scientific knowledge and describes exemplary care of older people. The inclusion of evidence-based and outcome-based practices throughout the book ensures that all readers, be they novices or experts, will have a reliable and beneficial reference to guide their practice.

The authors are from a number of countries, and the content of each chapter is presented generically to ensure international applicability. Each author is a recognised expert in his or her subject area, and all present their topics with a focus that is practical, rather than academic.

The goal of the book is to assist nurses in the provision of practical contemporary holistic care for older people. The underlying theme of the book is to stress the concepts of 'caring' and 'dignity'.

About the Authors

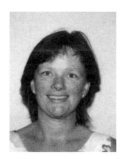

Catherine Barrett
Chapter 9

Catherine Barrett is a doctoral candidate with the School of Nursing at the University of Melbourne (Australia). Catherine has more than 20 years of experience in aged-care nursing—including the management of a residential-care unit and work as an external auditor for the Aged Care Standards and Accreditation Agency. Catherine has worked with the National Ageing Research Institute on several projects related to falls prevention. She is a co-director of Desirable Outcomes Pty Ltd, a business committed to promoting sexual and sensual health for adults in aged care and disability services.

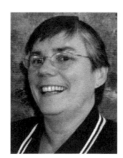

Elizabeth Beattie
Chapter 11

Elizabeth Beattie, PhD, RN, is currently a member of the research faculty at the School of Nursing, and project director of the Wandering Behavior Research Team, University of Michigan (USA). She has an extensive clinical and educational background in psychogeriatric nursing gained in Australia, the UK, and the USA, and has worked with individuals with dementia, their families, and caregivers since 1982. Elizabeth's research focus is wandering behaviour related to dementia, and her current research is on the impact of wandering on functional abilities, such as eating, in nursing-home residents.

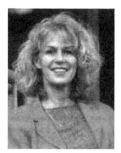

Susan Carmody
Subject Specialist Editor

Susan Carmody has been a nurse for more than thirty years. After her hospital-based training and having gained extensive clinical experience, Susan moved into management and quality assurance and commenced her own business, 'Health Force', which assists hospitals and other health organisations achieve the highest nursing standards and accreditation through education and quality improvement. In the past ten years Susan has concentrated her management and quality-control expertise on community aged care. She gains her greatest satisfaction from seeing her nursing colleagues come up with new ideas, be motivated to study and gain qualifications, and take risks to better themselves and achieve their personal and professional goals.

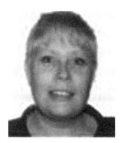

Eddi Cohen
Chapter 3

Eddi Cohen is a registered nurse and an international speaker and author who divides her time between between Sydney (Australia) and Los Angeles (USA). Her wide-ranging interests include nosocomial infections and hygiene practices, critical care, emergency and aviation medicine, violence and aggression in health care, terrorism, disaster management, and critical incident stress. Eddi has been consulting, writing, and teaching in Australia for more than ten years. She is presently medical director of Mobile Medical Systems International (Australia) and clinical nurse consultant with EMS Network International (USA). She also serves as director of training for AIRescue International, a Los Angeles-based air medical retrieval service.

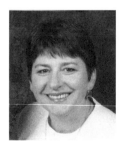

Keren Day
Chapter 8

Keren Day is a continence nurse consultant of more than 15 years experience. She currently is working at Ballarat Health Services (Victoria, Australia) in a regional, community-based, multidisciplinary continence service. Her experience includes management of a community-nursing continence service, coordination of the Victorian Continence Resource Centre, and establishment of a new multidisciplinary continence service. Keren has been involved in government working committees to develop continence services at both state and federal levels. More recently she has undertaken clinical research in the objective assessment of constipation in the elderly in residential care and in development of best-practice in bowel management.

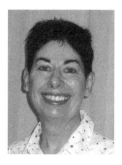

Robyn Dealtry

Chapter 13

Robyn Dealtry is a registered nurse who spent nine years in Singapore in the 1970s where she raised a family and worked with a Singapore private nurses' agency. After returning to Australia, Robyn worked in gerontic nursing and post-anaesthesia nursing. She established the Acute Pain Service at Westmead Hospital (Sydney, Australia) and is now the clinical nurse consultant and team leader of that service. Robyn has spoken at many local, national, and international conferences and, in collaboration with the College of Nursing (New South Wales, Australia), wrote the first distance-education package in assessing and managing acute adult pain. Robyn has written two journal articles on the management of trauma pain and a book chapter on epidural pain management. Robyn also holds a position on the editorial board of *South-East Asian Cardiothoracic Nurses Journal*. Robyn specialises in acute postoperative, trauma, and advanced cancer pain management.

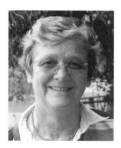

Sue Forster

Subject Specialist Editor; Chapters 1, 2, 15, and 20

Sue Forster completed her general nurse training in the Queen Alexandra Royal Naval Nursing Service in the UK and abroad. She has extensive clinical, educational, and managerial experience at senior levels gained from a long nursing career in Europe, Australia, and Africa. For the past ten years Sue has managed her own educational consultancy business. Her special interests include gerontic care, continuous quality improvement, and human-resource management. Sue is dedicated to the education and empowerment of her nursing colleagues through the provision of sound evidence-based practice within a holistic framework of quality care.

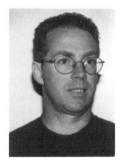

Keith Hill

Chapter 9

Keith Hill is a physiotherapist with more than 20 years of experience in rehabilitation and aged care. Keith's PhD thesis was entitled 'Balance studies in older people', and he has published numerous papers in this area. Keith is a senior research fellow at the National Ageing Research Institute and co-director of the falls and balance clinic at the Melbourne Extended Care and Rehabilitation Service (Victoria, Australia). He was recently project manager for a successful multifactorial, multidisciplinary falls-prevention project in residential aged care.

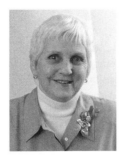

Rosalie Hudson

Chapter 14

Dr Rosalie Hudson's varied nursing and theological career is now focused on aged care and palliative care. As an aged-care consultant she explores end-of-life issues for people in residential aged care, and as an author, teacher, and associate professor with the University of Melbourne (Australia) she seeks to raise the profile of gerontic nursing. Rosalie has presented and published numerous papers and articles internationally on the subjects of spirituality, palliative care, dementia, pastoral care, and ethics at the end of life. She has co-authored two books on death and dying, and has contributed chapters to several other Ausmed publications. Rosalie has had 12 years' experience as a director of nursing of a 50-bed nursing home and, more recently, has served as the Victorian project officer for the Australian Palliative Aged Care Project. She enjoys family life with her husband, adult children, and grandchildren.

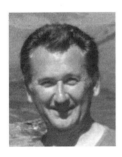

Graham A. Jackson

Chapter 12

Dr Graham A. Jackson is a consultant psychiatrist in Glasgow (Scotland). He is also an honorary lecturer at the Dementia Services Development Centre at Stirling University and is co-author, with Dr Alan Jacques of the book *Understanding Dementia*. Graham has been involved in research into behaviour problems in dementia and has published numerous papers on the subject. Before training in psychiatry, Graham was a general medical practitioner.

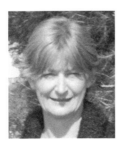

Sandra Keppich-Arnold

Chapter 16

Sandra Keppich-Arnold is a registered psychiatric nurse with postgraduate qualifications in health education. She has been involved in community aged psychiatry for the past 15 years and has contributed to the establishment of a number of innovative community treatment and consultancy services aimed at improving outcomes for people with dementia and delirium. Sandra has been particularly interested in ensuring that nurses and others approach dementia care positively, and she has been actively involved in a number of action groups to highlight the issues pertinent to improved dementia management. Sandra is an associate director of nursing and coordinator of the Mobile Aged Psychiatry Service at Caulfield General Medical Centre (Melbourne, Australia).

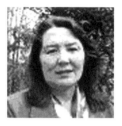

Linda Kilworth
Chapter 6

Linda Kilworth is a dietitian nutritionist who has worked for more than twelve years as a consultant to various chains of residential-care facilities in Brisbane and south-east Queensland (Australia). Her main role is to advise on nutritional management and dietary planning for the residential aged-care populations and on food-service management and standards generally. Linda is involved in writing and developing policies and procedures, communicating these to the relevant staff members, and developing processes of review and evaluation. This consultancy also encompasses call-outs to various residential aged-care facilities to conduct individual dietary assessments and prescription, to develop nutrition screening methods, and to provide practical advice on dietary modifications.

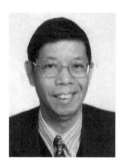

Alex Yui-huen Kwan
Chapters 19 and 21

Alex Yui-huen Kwan is a professor at the Department of Applied Social Studies, City University of Hong Kong. He is an active researcher in the gerontology field, and has published journal articles on elderly suicide, elderly abuse, attitudes towards older people, caregiver behaviour, and comparative studies on ageing. Alex is the author of several books (mainly in Chinese) on the social and psychological care of the aged, and has also edited several practical work manuals and training manuals on these subjects.

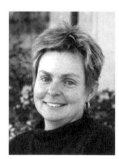

Melissa Lindeman
Chapter 9

Melissa Lindeman has qualifications in social science, policy studies, and adult education. Before joining the National Ageing Research Institute (NARI, Melbourne, Australia) in 1998, she was employed by the Victorian Department of Human Services in the Aged Care Branch. In her role as a research fellow in NARI's Public Health Division, she worked on a diverse range of projects many of which had a focus on education and workforce development. She joined the Batchelor Institute of Indigenous Tertiary Education as senior lecturer in allied health in 2003.

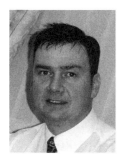

Colin MacDonald
Chapter 12

Colin MacDonald is a registered general and mental-health nurse. He is the charge nurse of a 30-bed long-stay hospital ward for people with dementia who have challenging behaviour. The ward is situated in Bonnybridge Hospital (Scotland)—a small community hospital for older people. Colin also works on a part-time basis with the Dementia Services Development Centre (DSDC) at Stirling University (Scotland) as an associate trainer in delivering training sessions on dementia and challenging behaviour. In 1997 Colin completed a research pilot study questioning the use of antipsychotic drugs in the care and treatment of people with dementia, and this led to the publication of 'Who's in Control?' (MacDonald & Teven 1997, DSDC, Stirling University).

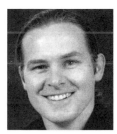

Hylton Menz
Chapter 5

Hylton Menz graduated with a bachelor's degree in podiatry from La Trobe University (Victoria, Australia) in 1993, and more recently completed his PhD at the Prince of Wales Medical Research Institute (New South Wales, Australia) investigating gait patterns in older people. He has worked as a lecturer at La Trobe University and the University of Western Sydney (New South Wales, Australia). Hylton is currently NHMRC Australian Clinical Research Fellow at the Musculoskeletal Research Centre at La Trobe University.

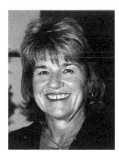

Patsy Montgomery
Chapter 7

Pasty Montgomery is a registered nurse, registered midwife, and stomal therapist who holds a degree in education from Monash University (Melbourne, Australia). She is co-founder of the Gastrostomy Information Support Service (GISS), president of the Peninsula Ostomy Association (Melbourne), and coordinator and clinical nurse consultant for the Abbott Nutrition Service (Victoria, Australia). Patsy provides a support service for tube-fed patients following discharge from hospital into the community, and also provides advice and support for the families and carers of patients. This includes information and help for managing enteral tubes and equipment, advice about methods of feeding and nursing care, and information regarding supply of formula, equipment, and pumps. She also organises in-service training, workshops, videos, and literature for healthcare professionals in these areas.

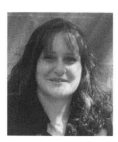

Letitia Quirk
Chapter 18

Having completed her general nurse training at the Mercy Hospital, Young (NSW, Australia), Letitia Quirk worked in both private and public hospitals as well as in a busy medical centre, before entering the aged-care sector. She was introduced to the benefits of lavender by a diversional therapist and personally witnessed its calming effect on residents. Letitia then developed an interest in natural therapies and went on to complete diplomas and certificates in remedial massage, natural therapies aromatherapy, and reflexology. Letitia is a member of the Holistic Nurses Association of NSW and has served on the education subcommittee of the Australian College of Holistic Nurses. She lectures at the NSW College of Nursing on complementary therapies and is a tutor at the Multiversity School of Natural Therapies (Burwood, Sydney, Australia), as well as acting as a consultant in complementary therapies to aged-care facilities and other healthcare facilities. Letitia is currently the deputy director of nursing at Veronica Nursing Home, Kincumber (NSW).

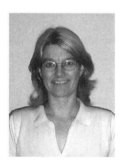

Robyn Smith
Chapter 9

Robyn Smith is an experienced public health researcher, and an aged-care occupational therapist. She currently manages the development of allied health research for Northern Health and was formerly the director of public health at the National Ageing Research Institute (both in Melbourne, Australia). Her main research interests focus on fostering sustainable change and the application of research evidence in health and residential aged-care.

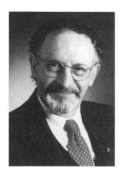

Geoff Sussman
Chapter 17

Geoff Sussman is a pharmacist. He is a graduate of the Victorian College of Pharmacy, member of the Pharmaceutical Society of Australia, member of the Society of Hospital Pharmacists, and associate fellow of the Australian Institute of Pharmacy Management. He is currently a senior lecturer in the Department of Pharmacy Practice, Monash University (Victoria, Australia). Geoff has vast experience in clinical pharmacy, clinical research, and product evaluation, and has published widely on the topic. For 15 years he was the director of Pharmacy Services at the Repatriation General Hospital (Melbourne, Australia). Geoff has lectured extensively on drugs and pharmacology for many years. He is an associate of the National Ageing Research Institute (Melbourne, Australia).

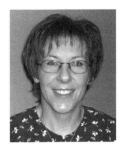

Sue Templeton
Chapter 4

Sue Templeton has extensive experience in the management of acute and chronic wounds. She is a clinical nurse consultant specialising in advanced wound care with the Royal District Nursing Service of South Australia, a clinical tutor with the University of Adelaide (Australia), and an active member of several professional organisations. Sue previously held the position of clinical lecturer with the University of Adelaide (Australia) and she was the clinical nurse consultant in the Department of Plastic and Reconstructive Surgery at Royal Adelaide Hospital for several years. As well as participating in the development of wound and Doppler competencies, Sue has participated in the development of a clinical pathway for management of venous leg ulcers, developed wound-assessment tools, and been active in policy development in wound management. She has presented at local and national forums and frequently conducts education sessions for nurses in a variety of settings. In 2002 Sue was awarded the South Australian Nursing Excellence Award in the category of Community Registered Nurse.

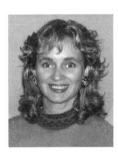

Lynn Varcin-Coad
Chapter 10

Lynn Varcin-Coad is a physiotherapist and Feldenkrais practitioner who has her own consultancy business, 'Manual Handling Systems'. As a result of her professional experience and studies (including her master's degree which researched the topic of spinal loads while repositioning people in wheelchairs), Lynn has developed a unique concept for manual handling. This combines freestyle-lifting training, body awareness, and competency-based training for adult workers in aged care and community services. Lynn has produced manual-handling videos and training packages independently and in conjunction with the Home and Community Services Resource Unit of Queensland (Australia). She is also a sessional lecturer for the faculty of Nursing and Health and the faculty of Physiotherapy and Exercise Science at Griffith University (Queensland, Australia).

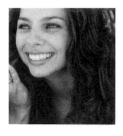

Jacie-Lee Whitfield
Chapter 22

Jacie-Lee Whitfield has been actively involved in aged care for many years, and has served in a wide variety of roles—including nursing assistant, domestic worker, food-service attendant, diversional therapist, administration officer, and coordinator. To complement her wide practical experience, Jacie has completed tertiary education in applied ethics, justice administration, psychology, health management, and Spanish. In 1999, she launched her own consultancy business, Jacie-Lee Consulting, and has since worked with many organisations, assisting them to achieve accreditation and to comply with occupational health-and-safety legislation.

Chapter 1

Nursing Older People

Sue Forster

Introduction

Nursing older people, or gerontic nursing, is now recognised as a specialised area of nursing. The word 'gerontic' is derived from the Greek word *geron*, meaning 'old man' or 'old age', and courses in gerontology are now widely available at undergraduate and postgraduate levels in institutes of higher education throughout the world. Such courses provide the theoretical basis for effective, evidence-based care of older people. Care of older people is the underpinning tenet of this book.

The sciences of medicine, nursing, nutrition, and environmental studies, among others, have brought about a significant prolongation of life, especially in the past hundred years. 'Life expectancy, measured as the mean number of years to death for a defined group . . . increased significantly over the twentieth century' (Gray et al. 2000, p. 1). Because people are living longer, the aged population has expanded remarkably, and will continue to do so. Along with a decrease in mortality (and an increase in the aged population), there has been a significant increase in morbidity. This means that there is a greater number of frail and ill elderly people than ever before, and older people's specialist nurses are in high demand.

Institutionalised care in Care Homes is a specialty within the field of care of older people. However, health and social policy for older people in the UK prefers care to be provided within the home environments where possible. Non-institutionalised care of frail older people is often referred to as 'community care', and this is another specialty subject under the umbrella of gerontic care (Cluning 2001).

In any community, older people are its 'living historians', and they should be afforded the respect that they have earned through their roles in society. To provide proper respect and care, older people's nurses require knowledge and skills. In the past, members of pre-literate societies imparted knowledge and skills by communicating with each other through story-telling and anecdotes. In the modern world, the education of nurses is dominated by documented historical data and research results. But the sharing of stories, accumulated wisdom, and practical skills continues to play an important part in a truly rounded education. Specialist older people's nurses combine their theoretical knowledge with their shared wisdom and applied practical skills to ensure the dignity of the elderly through true *caring*. This book contributes to such empowerment through knowledge.

> 'Older people are the community's 'living historians', and they should be afforded the respect that they have earned.'

Knowledge base

Specialist older people's nurses need to apply their knowledge of both 'normal' and 'abnormal' ageing if they are to achieve optimal care of older people. The principle that 'structure is directly related to function' can be applied to the anatomical changes that take place during the ageing and disease processes, and to the consequential physiological alterations that follow.

Ageing, chronological and physiological, commences at conception and progresses through the stages of development, maturation, and degeneration. The use of the term 'old age' varies among societies. However, in most developed countries, it is used to describe people aged more than 65 years. At the age of 65 years, most people are expected to retire from the workforce and, in some jurisdictions, legislation deems them eligible for an aged pension. It is ironic that, as life expectancy increases, some governments are considering the introduction of 'age-neutral' policies to postpone the retirement of a diminishing workforce. In addition, as life expectancy increases, so is the overall degree of 'wellness', and to be forced to retire involuntarily while still fit and able to contribute can cause people to suffer financial, psychological, and physical problems.

It has been proposed that people should be classified as 'young-old' (those aged between 55 and 74 years) and 'old-old' (those aged 75 and over) (Neugarten 1970). The rationale for this proposed separation of the older population is that each group had different needs and 'life tasks' to achieve. Part of caring for older people involves ascertaining these needs and 'life tasks' for each person, and then implementing a plan of action that will assist each person to achieve his or her goals. Unfortunately, goals are not always achieved, but identifying and attempting to meet a person's goals should be the rationale in planning the care of every person.

> 'Identifying and attempting to meet a person's goals should be the rationale in planning the care of every person.'

Skills needed by nurses

Specialist older people's nurses must possess a plethora of skills if they are to plan and implement care for older people successfully. In so doing, nurses need to be accurate and efficient in applying the constructs of the nursing process. These are:

- assessment;
- analysis;
- planning;
- implementation; and
- evaluation.

The skills to do these things effectively must be of an exceedingly high standard because a large proportion of older people who require nursing care have organic or functional brain disorders that hamper effective cognition, thus making *assessment* of the person's needs more difficult. In addition, co-morbidity must also be taken into account when making nursing assessments.

Following assessment comes *analysis*, *planning*, and *implementation*. The planning and implementing of individualised, holistic care depends on accurate assessment in sometimes difficult circumstances, and the care plans that result should be prescriptive, individualised, and dynamic 'blueprints' for the whole healthcare team to follow.

The final stage of the process is *evaluation*. Every care plan should be evaluated. The nurse needs to use objective evaluative criteria to assess if the 'person-centred goals' have been met. Skills obtained from applying 'evidence-based practice' and 'outcome-based practice' methodologies can assist the nurse in the evaluation stage of the process.

To hone the skills required of an older people's specialist nurse, a combination of scientific data, intuitive analysis, and practical experience is needed. Application of these skills in the clinical setting promotes quality care and ensures dignity for older people in the final stages of their lives.

Each of these skills is considered in greater detail below, with particular reference to care provision in Care Homes.

The contructs of the nursing process

Specialist older people's nurses must possess a plethora of skills if they are to plan and implement care for older people successfully. In so doing, nurses need to be accurate and efficient in applying the constructs of the nursing process. These are:

- assessment;
- analysis;
- planning;
- implementation; and
- evaluation.

Assessment

Assessments must be meticulous if they are to be the linchpin of the care plan. Two requirements for achieving precise assessments are:

▶ teamwork; and
▶ efficient assessment tools.

A collaborative approach from the entire health *team* is needed if the assessment results are to be usefully employed. The team should consist of the older person, his or her relatives and friends (if appropriate), nurses and carers, doctors, and allied health professionals (for example, physiotherapists, nutritionists, occupational therapists, and speech pathologists).

Reliable and valid tools are also required to achieve accurate assessment results. These tools are usually documents in the form of questionnaires or forms that are designed to elicit pertinent information. Pertinent information that is required includes the person's physical, psychological, and social status. This three-dimensional approach is referred to as the 'biopsychosocial model'. This model, first developed by the psychiatrist Engel (1977), is readily adaptable to the needs of nurses and ensures an holistic evaluation of the person. A list of some of the assessments that should be completed in using this model can be found in Table 1.1 (below). Other models can also be used.

Table 1.1 Biopsychosocial model

Physical	Psychological	Social
Medical diagnosis	General well-being	Past history
Vital signs	Mental status	Support structure
Clinical manifestations	Cognitive ability	Family structure
(pain, wounds, etc.)	Behaviour patterns	Education
Neurological status	Spiritual needs	Religion
(special senses,	Sexual needs	Ethnicity
communication, etc.)	Beliefs and values	Cultural needs
Nutrition and	Emotional needs	Financial status
hydration status	Recreation activities	Leisure activities
Mobility status	Safety needs	Safety needs
Skin condition		
Continence status		

Author's creation

Because of the sheer volume of data required, and the need to include the older person and his or her representatives in care provision, some Care Homes are utilising pre-admission assessment tools. These tools are given to prospective residents to complete when they first approach the Care Home for placement. The completion of pre-admission assessments serves two objectives: (i) the person and his or her representatives are involved in completing the documents within a realistic time-frame; and (ii) the act of responding to questions is believed to assist the person to adapt to his or her impending relocation.

Analysis

The analysis of data requires a combination of scientific evidence, intuitive analysis, and knowledge gained through practical experience if an effective analysis is to be made.

There are many excellent examples of data analysis throughout this book. Each chapter author has provided suggestions for evidence-based practice within his or her own specialised subject area, and all of these proposed actions are ultimately based upon data analysis.

Planning of care

The compilation and formalisation of proposed actions is the substructure of care planning. A collaborative approach from the whole health team is needed if the care plan is to be of real value to the older person. However, in many Care Homes, the onerous task of formulating a care plan is often left to the nurses and carers.

In Care Homes the older people's specialist nurse is often the only qualified gerontic nurse on any given shift. Doctors may visit their patients on an 'as required' basis, and allied health professionals are employed on a casual basis or called in as a result of a specific referral. This situation leaves the planning of care to the nurse specialist and his or her team of carers. Input from the rest of the health care team is often spasmodic, fragmented, and untimely. The resulting care plan is generated on the basis of the specialist nurse's knowledge, clinical experience, and intuition. Depending upon the size of the Care Home, the design and implementation of an appropriate and efficient care plan can be very time-consuming, and the responsibility for care planning can thus place an inordinate amount of stress on the specialist nurse.

In an care setting an appropriate and efficient care plan should be person-centred and individualised. All unmet needs should be addressed by formulating a 'person-centred objective', followed by documentation of the specific prescriptions of care to be implemented. Review and evaluation dates should also be cited. Some institutional policies dictate the use of 'nursing diagnoses' to be included in their care plans, whereas others prefer a descriptive identification of the issue under examination to be recorded.

There are several computer programs available to assist nurses in formulating care plans. However, because of their generic nature, these programs are not suitable as a standard menu for all, and they must therefore be individualised to particular needs.

All entries on a care plan must be linked to the older person's assessment results. For example, if the assessment results indicate that the person is incontinent of urine, the issue should be noted as 'incontinent of urine', followed by a 'person-centred objective'—for example, 'Mrs W will be comfortable'. The next entries should direct the caregiver as to what actions are required to deal with the situation—for example, to change clothes when soiled, to clean perineal area after each episode, to use a nominated bed protector at night, and so on. Finally,

'All entries on a care plan must be linked to the aged person's assessment results.'

a review date should be nominated for when the objective and the corresponding actions will be evaluated.

Care provision

The older people's specialist nurse is professionally and legally responsible for care provision. Due to unplanned staff shortages in Care Homes, this nurse may be in the untenable situation of not only having to provide direct care, but also having to supervise the provision of care by a team of carers who are not always in the same physical location as the nurse supervisor. In the UK, National Minimum Standards for Care Homes for Older People, published under section 23(1) of The Care Standards Act (2000) specifies staffing ratios for UK Care Homes and any Care Home which fails to meet this may jeopardise their registration (Secretary of State for Health 2001).

> 'The older people's specialist nurse is professionally and legally responsible for care provision.'

Care provision is dictated not only by the older person's needs but also by the philosophy of the organisation. Ideally the philosophy, mission statement, vision statement, and organisational objectives should be formulated by all members of staff, and frequently reviewed. All of these documents should clearly identify the rationale for functioning as a Care Home for older people. The inclusive beliefs and values form a distinctive 'code of practice' for the Care Home, which can be made known to potential residents and future staff. New residents need to be able to make informed choices regarding their future home, and

> 'The inclusive beliefs and values form a distinctive 'code of practice' to be made known to potential residents and future staff.'

these choices should be based upon knowledge of care provision by the service. Similarly, new employees should be equal partners in the staff-selection process, and should be able to evaluate if they are ethically attuned with the organisation.

Too often, a philosophical statement does not reflect the ethos and objectives of the specific organisation, and is merely a duplication of the manifesto of another facility. An organisation's philosophy, mission statement, vision statement, and objectives should reflect all of the following:

- the value of older people (and their entitlements);
- employees' beliefs and values;
- the rights of the residents (dignity, confidentiality, choices, freedom, and so on);
- care provision (including standards of care);
- expectations and outcomes of care;
- what the service specialises in, and what it cannot provide;
- inclusiveness (that is, who is included in care provision); and
- contract arrangements.

Care provision should be exactly that—'providing care'. Nurses and carers need to be competent at their tasks and skills, and management needs to ensure that safe staff/resident ratios exist, and that all necessary equipment is provided to achieve optimal physical and psychological comfort for each person. In some situations it might be necessary to refer people to specialist services (for example, psychologists, social workers, or mental-health personnel) or to transfer them to hospitals for appropriate care provision.

Models of care

Many facilities find that the use of a model of care, or a combination of models, enables them to meet most residents' needs within the resources of the Care Home. Such models of care have been formulated on the basis of years of clinical 'trial and error' and research findings. The selection of a particular model depends upon the assessment results (including medical diagnosis) of each older person. Each model has its merits, and each should be evaluated for its efficacy with each resident.

Whichever model is used, it is necessary for all staff members to familiarise themselves with that model. On any shift within a facility, the combinations and permutations of staff members (for example, the ratio of novice employees to experienced staff members) are never exactly the same. Without sound knowledge of the model and avoidance of 'team-splitting', the outcomes are likely to be less than favourable.

The model should be judged using the evaluation criteria of 'evidence-based practice' and 'outcome-based practice'. People benefit from the process only if the model is applied as it was intended to be applied.

Evaluation

The final stage (but not the end stage) of the nursing process is evaluation. Evaluation is synonymous with assessment, which makes the nursing process a never-ending cyclical procedure. From any evaluation, the need for more assessments emerges; these assessments, in turn, require more interventions and further evaluation.

Ideally evaluation of an outcome should be based upon measurable, objective, valid criteria. However, this is not always possible, and subjective, norm-referenced criteria are the only reliable tools available to the assessor. Table 1.2 (below) illustrates a care plan entry, and Table 1.3 (below) illustrates corresponding evaluative criteria.

Table 1.2 care plan entry

Issue	Objective	Actions	Review
Incontinent of urine	Mrs W will be comfortable	Change clothes when soiled Clean perineal area after each episode Use large pad and net pants at night	1 June

Note: The actual care plan would include date, signature, name, and status of author

Author's creation

Table 1.3 Evaluative criteria

Measurable, objective, valid	Subjective, norm-referenced
Clothes clean and dry Perineal area clean and dry Perineal area not red or excoriated Mrs W is not gesturing discomfort Large pad and pants worn at night	Mrs W states that she is comfortable She is in the same condition as all other residents Her bed linen is the same as all other residents

Author's creation

On the date of review, a corresponding entry should be included in the person's notes noting whether the person-centred objective was met or unmet (citing the evaluative criteria utilised). Accurate documentation is the only method that can ensure that future care plans are not repetitions of previous failed attempts. If something has been ineffective in the past it is likely to be ineffective in the future. In contrast, if there is accurate documentary evidence that certain actions were effective, future successes are almost guaranteed.

Conclusion

The stigma attached to nursing older people is slowly being eroded by the high quality of care provided, the ever-expanding knowledge base, the availability of extensive research findings, and the increased self-esteem of older people's specialist nurses themselves.

It was once stated that older people nurses were 'somewhat inferior in capabilities or not good enough for acute settings or ready to "go to pasture"' (Eliopoulos 1987, pp 12–13). This is certainly not the case today, and most older people's specialist nurses are highly qualified, highly motivated, and exemplary nurse practitioners who often work under duress. They gain their rewards from the knowledge that they provide high-quality nursing and dignity to those in their care.

> 'Older people's nurses gain their rewards from the knowledge that they provide high-quality nursing and dignity to those in their care.'

Chapter 2

Nursing Assessments

Sue Forster

Introduction

Assessments are an essential prerequisite to caring for frail and ill older people. In the UK, formal assessment of continuing care need is required for: (i) placement in Care Homes; (ii) review at the time of transfer; and (iii) review at stipulated intervals thereafter on an ongoing basis. Health and social care assessments result thus facilitate the placement of an older person in a suitable 'fit-for-purpose' facility. The continuing care assessments assist with the planning, implementing, and adjusting of care provision once the resident has been admitted, as they form baseline information for the Care Home. Continuing care assessments are carried out by the NHS and local authorities.

When a person is admitted to a Care Home, the Care Home registered nurse is responsible for ongoing local nursing assessment. In most Care Homes, doctors visit their patients on an 'as-needed' basis and allied health professionals are either employed on a casual basis or are called in as a result of a specific referral. This situation means that the assessment of the person is co-ordinated by the nurse specialist and his or her team of carers. Input from the rest of the healthcare team may be spasmodic, fragmented, and untimely. It is therefore expedient for facilities to have policies, procedures, and clear guidelines in place to assist nurses in completing the assessment process efficiently and effectively.

There are numerous assessment software packages on the market to assist nurses with all of their documentation requirements, and if a package is selected wisely it can be an efficient time-saver that is of economic benefit to the organisation. When selecting a documentary package, consideration should be given to the package's applicability to the specific facility—in particular, whether its content reflects contemporary practice, and whether it meets legislative requirements.

The nature of assessment

Assessment involves the gathering of data relating to a person's physical, psychological, and social status before admission, at the time of admission, and following admission. This gathering of data involves interviewing the person (and his or her nominated representatives), physically assessing the person, and documenting the findings.

The procedure takes time and can be stressful for the person. Because older people are often sceptical about authority figures seeking information, it is important that the process not be too formal. This scepticism can be increased if the older person is reluctant to provide personal information to a younger person. A younger person in an apparent position of authority, especially one who reads questions from a structured questionnaire, can be interpreted by the older person as being impersonal, intrusive, or impertinent. To avoid these sorts of difficulties a more informal approach is often helpful, and much information can be gleaned from casual communication and observations while settling the person into his or her room, or during other interactions throughout the day.

> 'A younger person in a position of authority can be interpreted by the older person as being impersonal, intrusive, or impertinent.'

Once the data have been gathered through a combination of formal and informal means, one of the skills of assessment is collation of the information and presentation of the findings in a comprehensive and logical schema. This schema is the foundation upon which the planning of care is based, and if the schema is incomplete, the care plan will be inadequate. An inadequate care plan is like an unfinished jigsaw puzzle; in both cases the complete picture relies on guesswork. If guesswork is to be eliminated from care planning, thorough and complete assessments are needed.

Beginning an assessment

Assessment begins when the first contact is made. As soon as the person arrives at the Care Home, a subjective appraisal commences, and this continues until these initial impressions are proved or disproved on more formal assessment. It is important that assessments address only pertinent issues, and that they do not involve requesting information already received. Asking for information that has already been provided can cause frustration to older people, and can result in a breakdown of meaningful dialogue.

The assessor should take advantage of the fact that family and/or friends usually accompany the older person during admission. With the person's consent, this is an opportunity to involve his or her representatives in the assessment process. These representatives can provide much information that would otherwise be undetected. Representatives can also sometimes correct misperceptions or 'fill in' forgotten details.

Assessing the whole person

As previously noted, if the 'jigsaw picture' assembled from the assessment is incomplete, guesswork is required and accurate analysis becomes very difficult. Assessments should therefore cover the 'whole person'.

In the past, assessments were usually limited to clinical manifestations of physical problems, with scant attention being paid to the person's psychological and social needs. Indeed, it was not until the 1970s that the 'social' parameter became part of the standard assessment process (Engel 1977). Contemporary practices now assess the whole person—including physical, psychological, and social status—rather than assessing only the person's physical status. Such assessment of the whole person requires the assessor to utilise an holistic framework.

Frameworks for assessment

Numerous assessment frameworks are available for the assessor to use. Indeed, it sometimes seems that there are as many frameworks as there are doctrines of care expounded by the many nurse theorists who have undertaken research projects! Three models that can be used as assessment frameworks are the biophysical model (shown in Figure 2.1, below), the systems model (Figure 2.2, below), and the needs model (Figure 2.3, below).

Physical	Psychological	Social
Medical diagnosis	General well-being	Past history
Vital signs	Mental status	Support structure
Clinical manifestations	Cognitive ability	Family structure
(pain, wounds, etc.)	Behaviour patterns	Education
Neurological status (special	Spiritual needs	Religion
senses, communication, etc.)	Sexual needs	Ethnicity
Nutrition and hydration status	Beliefs and values	Cultural needs
Mobility status	Emotional needs	Financial status
Skin condition	Recreation activities	Leisure activities
Continence status	Safety needs	Safety needs

Figure 2.1 Biopsychosocial model
Author's creation, adapted from Engel (1977)

System	Needs
Cardiovascular system	Nutrition
Endocrine system	Elimination
Gastrointestinal system	Sensory
Integumentary system	Communication
Musculoskeletal system	Continence
Nervous system	Hygiene
Respiratory system	Safety
Sensory system	. Sexuality
Urogenital system	Rest and sleep
	Comfort

Figure 2.2 Systems model
Author's creation

	Mobility

Figure 2.3 Needs model
Author's creation

Additional assessments that should be undertaken are shown in Figure 2.4 (below). Some of the criteria shown in Figure 2.4 could well be already included in the models noted previously, but nurses should ensure that the criteria listed in Figure 2.4 are included in any complete assessment.

Physical examination	Investigations	Psychosocial assessments
Height Weight Temperature Pulse Respiratory rate Blood pressure	Blood analysis Urinalysis X-rays and scans	Mini-mental examination Depression rating scale Substance usage

Figure 2.4 Additional assessments
Author's creation

Assessment methods

Although there are many methods and tools available to assist nurses with the assessment process, accurate results are dependent upon the knowledge and skills of the assessor. Effective interpersonal skills in association with a broad knowledge base are essential in obtaining valid data. Vision, hearing, smell, and touch are the most inexpensive and effective assessment tools. Assessment methods are categorised in Figure 2.5 (below).

History	Physical examination	Test
Asking questions Active listening	Examination Observations Measuring vital signs Noting odours	Conducting tests Special investigations

Figure 2.5 Assessment methods
Author's creation

Before commencing any formal assessment procedures, a detailed explanation should be given to the person and any representatives who are present. This explanation should be in plain (non-technical) language and should focus on obtaining informed consent from the person. An interpreter might be required to obtain informed consent from people who are 'culturally and linguistically different' (CALD).

A private area should be used to maintain dignity and ensure confidentiality. Other issues that should be addressed are lighting, temperature, comfortable chairs, comfort supplies (for example, fluids, snacks, tissues), and ensuring that no interruptions occur.

All necessary prosthetic devices (such as spectacles, hearing aids, and dentures) should be in use. Before beginning the assessment, nurses should ensure that these prosthetic devices are well maintained and functional. Spectacles should be clean and of the right type (for example, reading glasses should be available if required). Hearing aids should be working well—with a snugly fitting earpiece and charged batteries. Dentures should be clean and comfortable. Any other appropriate communication aids should be available (for example, pictures, alphabet boards, or tactile cues).

It is important that the assessor is aware of any previous information received by the facility, and that he or she checks that it is accurate. The current assessment should augment this information, rather than needlessly reiterating questions that have already been answered.

Throughout the discussion, the nurse should be alert for any signs of fatigue or discomfort in the elderly person. If these are noted, the interview should be curtailed. It is often necessary to conduct an assessment over an extended time (perhaps weeks), rather than all at once.

Assessment domains

Any complete assessment should include all three assessment domains—physical, psychological, and social. In assessing these domains, nurses should be cognisant of the numerous changes that occur with ageing.

In the *physical domain*, nurses should be aware of the insidious nature of the anatomical and physiological changes that accompany normal ageing. Every system of the body deteriorates in its metabolic function—at both the microscopic level and the macroscopic level (Holmes 1999).

In the *psychological domain*, nurses should be aware that older persons might have a distorted perception of their situation (Holmes 1997), which can be related either to the ageing process or to disease processes.

Finally, in the *social domain*, nurses should be aware that older people have often 'out-lived' many of their family members and friends. Their support networks are frequently located in their communities—such as neighbours, social groups, and clubs (Cluning 2001). A lack of live-in support networks means that the aged population all too commonly experiences social isolation, grief, loneliness, and depression.

Physical domain

The physical domain is probably the easiest domain to assess—because there is an expectation that doctors and nurses 'poke, prod, measure, and test' those in their care. The person therefore often takes a passive role in these procedures. However, although many people enjoy the attention bestowed upon them, some people can become restive (or even hostile). If a person does become uncomfortable or agitated, it is advisable to desist and try again later.

Information that should be gathered in relation to the physical domain includes:

▶ a full health history;
▶ a statement of the person's general well-being;
▶ a full review of each system (see Figure 2.2, page 14);
▶ clinical manifestations;
▶ medical diagnosis;
▶ vital signs;
▶ sensory deficits;
▶ weight-to-height ratio;
▶ laboratory results (haematology, biochemistry, urinalysis);
▶ other test results (X-rays, scans); and
▶ treatment regimens (including medicines).

Assessment alert in the physical domain

Assessors should be aware of factors that might influence information collected during assessment of the physical domain. It is important to realise that:

• a person's fear of the prognosis can influence his or her responses;
• altered mental status can impede provision of accurate information;
• pain can be underreported due to reduced sensitivity (or greater tolerance) to pain in older people;
• the 'normal' ranges given for vital signs are based upon all adults, *not* specifically elderly adults;
• sensory deficits are present in all older people to varying degrees;
• the person might be attending ongoing specialist appointments; and
• the resident might be taking various 'over-the-counter' and complementary medications (in addition to known prescribed medicines).

Psychological domain

The psychological domain is quite often the most difficult domain to assess. Many people consider that the information being sought is of a private nature that has nothing to do with the doctors or nurses. An explanation of why the information is needed and the purpose for which it is to be used can allay some of the person's fears, but sometimes no amount of explanation can alter deeply entrenched beliefs.

Information that should be gathered in relation to the psychological domain includes:

▶ a full mental-health history;
▶ a statement of the resident's mental well-being;
▶ a list of concerns;
▶ cognitive ability (including educational achievements);
▶ communication (languages spoken or understood, preferred language, primary language);
▶ test results (mini-mental examination, depression-rating scale, behaviour patterns, rest and sleep patterns);
▶ personal likes and dislikes (including beliefs and values, emotional needs, sexual needs, spiritual needs, safety needs);
▶ substance use (alcohol, tobacco, medicines); and
▶ terminal wishes.

Assessment alert in the psychological domain

Assessors should be aware of factors that might influence information collected during assessment of the psychological domain. It is important to realise that:

• older people are sometimes reserved;
• a significant proportion of institutionalised older persons are clinically depressed;
• people with dementia often revert to their primary languages;
• elderly people consider some subjects taboo (especially those related to sexuality);
• some beliefs are held covertly;
• substance abuse might be denied; and
• some people have an irrational fear of death.

Social domain

The social domain (like the physical domain) is another relatively easy domain to assess because people usually consider that most of the information being gathered is virtually 'public knowledge'. They therefore do not feel unduly threatened in being asked to provide the details. Information that needs to be gathered in relation to the social domain includes:

▶ a social history or profile;
▶ support networks (family, friends, pets, clubs and organisations);
▶ significant relationships;

- religious or spiritual needs;
- cultural, racial, or ethnic needs;
- recreation, leisure activities, or hobbies;
- financial status; and
- legal issues (guardianship, will, funeral arrangements).

Assessment alert in the social domain

Assessors should be aware of factors that might influence information collected during assessment of the social domain. It is important to realise that:
- residents often don't like to state their 'favourites' for fear of sanctions;
- pet ownership and care is of paramount concern;
- religious and spiritual beliefs gain more importance towards the end of life; and
- financial matters are often considered private.

Functional assessments

Functional assessments are an appraisal of what residents can and cannot do for themselves. The assessment should be limited to the activities of daily living (ADLs)—because it is impossible to examine every theoretical aspect of life.

An historical profile of the person can be of great assistance. The example of Elsie (Box, below) is a simple example of how an apparently significant finding can undergo reassessment when seen in its historical context. Only by comparing past and present known facts can the nurse determine the importance of an assessment result.

Elsie

An assessment of activities of daily living (ADLs) revealed that Elsie was unable to prepare meals for herself—a finding that the assessor initially felt was probably of some significance. However, upon examining Elsie's historical profile, it soon become apparent that Elsie had not been able to prepare her own meals for a very long time.

Nurse assessors can determine the importance of an assessment result only by comparing past and present known facts.

Duration of assessments

To analyse assessment results accurately, the data should be gathered over a period of time. The period of time required can be ascertained only retrospectively—once a pattern emerges. Longitudinal studies reveal patterns.

From these identified patterns, interventions can be planned for each person—as was the case with Maude (see Box, below).

Maude

Maude, a 92-year-old widow displayed agitation only on Friday evenings. The nursing staff attempted to discover whether Friday had some special significance for Maude. For example, they made enquiries about the day of her husband's death, but found that he had died on a Monday. Despite their best efforts, nurses could not discover the cause of Maude's distress every Friday evening.

Even though they never discovered the significance of Fridays, the establishment of a definite pattern was very helpful. When staff members provided extra attention in the form of sitting and playing cards with Maude every Friday evening, her agitation diminished. As long as she had company and was participating in something she enjoyed, Maude's distress was not overtly manifested.

Sometimes patterns can be identified after a few days (for example, urinary continence), but others can take months (for example, dysfunctional behaviour associated with a full moon). Whatever the case might be, it is only by establishing routines that reflect the person's usual patterns that a satisfactory outcome can be achieved.

Conclusion

Assessments are an invasion into a person's life. The assessor must appreciate that the assessment procedure can be quite stressful for the person and his or her representatives. Assessment can be stressful to the *person involved* because, apart from the stress of the procedure itself, it represents a need for assistance during the remainder of the person's life; and it is stressful to the *person's representatives* because they have to accept that they alone can no longer care for their loved one. Both parties grieve their loss.

> 'Effective communication and skilful assessment maintain the dignity of all those who are involved in the assessment process.'

Effective communication and skilful assessment not only gather the data needed to plan care, but also maintain the dignity of all those who are involved in the assessment process.

Chapter 3

Skin and Oral Hygiene

Eddi Cohen

Introduction

The skin is the first line of defence in protecting the body from the environment, abuse, trauma, neglect, and infection. Apart from its role in protection, the skin is involved in sensation, metabolism, and thermoregulation.

Factors that influence the skin's normal flora (microorganisms that inhibit growth of harmful microbes) include age, nutritional status, and the environment. These factors, together with underlying illness, can also alter a person's susceptibility to disease.

The outermost layer of the skin has an *acid mantle* with a pH of 4.5–6.0 that retards bacterial and fungal growth, and that provides a barrier to prevent fluid and electrolyte loss. This acid mantle is made up of sebum (secreted from the sebaceous glands) and dead skin cells, and has a thin surface film that provides lubrication and hydration. Keratin, a major component of the epidermis, acts as waterproofing and minimises fluid loss through the epidermis.

Skin damage

Frequent bathing with alkaline cleansers such as soaps (which can have pH levels as high as 12), can dry the skin by removing the sebum, thus reducing the natural antimicrobial activity of the acid mantle and diminishing its protective properties. Soap is difficult to rinse off and remains behind on the skin. Depending on length of exposure, the skin can take up to 18 hours to return to its normal pH after being cleansed with traditional soap (Ayliffe, Collins & Taylor 1985). Even with normal washing using a limited amount of soap, a return to normal pH can take 45 minutes (Bryant & Rolstad 2001). In contrast, synthetic surfactants (often referred to as 'soap-free' cleansing alternatives) have pH levels closer to that of the normal acid mantle, and are easier to rinse off.

Intact skin is the first line of defence against infection. If violated, this creates a portal of entry for infection. Loss of surface moisture can lead to dry, itchy, flaky, scaling, and cracked skin—which leaves the tissue more susceptible to pressure breakdown and complicates healing. The maintenance of healthy skin is thus essential to the prevention of pressure sores and ulcers. If the integrity of the skin is compromised, this can result in ulcers, skin tears, dermatitis, abrasions, burns, erythema, and xerosis (dry skin). At least 70% of hospitalised patients and 90% of long-term Care Home residents have dry skin and are at risk of skin injury (Bryant & Rolstad 2001).

> 'At least 70% of hospitalised patients and 90% of long-term Care Home residents have dry skin and are at risk of skin injury.'

Ageing leads to increased nail thickness and decreased elasticity of the skin, with thinning of the dermis and flattening of the dermal–epidermal junction. Other risk factors for skin tears include sensory loss, poor nutritional status, impaired cognition, and dependency on others for activities of daily living.

Injuries to the skin can result from falls, bumping into objects, wheelchairs, bed-to-chair transfers, and rough handling of the skin—including the application of harsh soaps and cleansers and the use of rough washcloths and towels during hygiene care (McGough-Csarny & Kopac 1998). Because washcloths and towelling are important causes of skin tears, skin should always be 'patted dry', and never rubbed.

Evidence-based standards in skin care

Importance of bathing

Bathing is an important routine for comfort, infection control, and emotional well-being. However, many nurses do not consider bathing to be a technical 'clinical' procedure, and they often delegate it to health care assistants.

Evidence-based skin hygiene should be provided by trained staff members, and due attention should be given to proper procedure, assessment, and intervention. Optimal skin care washes away potentially dangerous microorganisms, protects the skin's normal flora and acid mantle, and ensures moisturisation.

Evidence-based guidelines for bathing

There is now significant research on which to establish evidence-based guidelines for bathing. These guidelines aim to maintain skin integrity and thus prevent pressure ulcers and skin tears in older people. The guidelines refer to the frequency of bathing, the cleansers used, and the abrasiveness and drag of washcloths employed in hygienic practices. Specific recommendations are listed in the Box below.

For more on evidence-based practice with respect to bathing, see 'Best practice in bathing', this chapter, page 27.

Evidence-based guidelines for skin care

Important evidence-based guidelines for good skin care include the following (AHCPR 1992):

- skin cleansing should occur at the time of soiling, and at routine intervals;
- frequency should be individualised according to patient needs and preferences;
- hot water should be avoided;
- mild cleansing agents that minimise irritation and dryness of the skin should be used;
- the force and friction applied to the skin during bathing should be minimised; and
- dry skin should be treated with moisturisers.

Friction

All surfactants, both natural cleansers and synthetic cleansers (detergents), clean by decreasing the surface tension. This allows debris (dirt) to be easily removed from the skin surface as matter is flushed away in showering and rinsing without excessive tissue damage.

Although friction is essential for effective cleaning, it should never be excessive. Excessive 'drag' on the epidermis can cause shearing, and thus create skin tears.

Frequency of bathing

Many older people do not need daily bathing. Older people commonly suffer from pruritic skin conditions, and constant itching and scratching can result in infections. Senile pruritus is experienced by 40% of older people, and this condition is strongly associated with frequency of bathing and the use of strong soaps (Frantz & Kinney 1986; Mason 1997).

Rather than full daily baths, 'top-and-tail' cleansing of the perineum, axillae, face and hands might be sufficient, allowing for such issues as incontinence and excessive sweating.

Incontinence

Incontinence among older people increases the risk of weakened and damaged skin. Moisture and poor skin hygiene can cause maceration of the skin, and colonisation with Gram-negative organisms can follow. Such organisms die on dry skin, but they proliferate in moist environments, such as damp skin folds.

A combination of incontinence and deep skin folds (such as those in the groin, axilla, under pendulous breasts, behind the scrotum, and other fat folds in obese persons) can predispose to such infection. More information on incontinence can be found later in this chapter (see 'Incontinence and moisture-related dermatitis', page 25).

Contaminated equipment

The equipment used in bathing can be a source of infection. Potable water can carry mycobacterium organisms, and basins (wet and dry) used for bed baths can be contaminated with Gram-negative bacteria and be responsible for outbreaks of infection on wards (Ayliffe, Collins & Taylor 1985). Contaminants can also be found in bar soaps, which become a medium for bacterial growth. This is why bar soaps have been prohibited in hospital settings as part of infection-control protocols (Kabara & Brady 1984).

'The equipment used in bathing can be a source of infection . . . potable water, basins (wet and dry), and bar soaps.'

Antimicrobial skin cleansers

Antimicrobial cleansing agents containing triclosan, chlorhexidine gluconate, and parachloroxylenol are not recommended for routine bathing—except for residents who are colonised with methicillin-resistant staphylococcus aureus

(MRSA). However, this is controversial because there is no evidence that regular use of an antimicrobial cleanser is effective (or necessary) in routine bathing. On the contrary, regular use of antimicrobial cleansers might give rise to drug-resistant organisms and suppress normal flora (Nix 2000).

Moisturisers

There are two main types of moisturisers:

▶ occlusives or *emollients*—such as petrolatum (petroleum jelly), dimethicone, or oils—which form an occlusive layer to prevent water from evaporating, and thus have a *softening effect* on the skin; and

▶ non-oily *humectants*—such as glycerin, propylene glycol, urea, and aloe—which improve the skin's moisture-binding capacity, thus having a *moisturising effect* on the skin.

Much misinformation exists about the use of glycerin as a skin moisturiser. Glycerin occurs as a natural by-product of soap-making, and is considered non-irritating and non-allergenic. There is also a synthetic version of glycerin (known as propylene glycol). The effects of glycerin with respect to moisture are directly proportional to the concentration of glycerin used in a particular product. The concentration of glycerin or propylene glycol in cosmetics, moisturisers, and other cosmetic grade products is such that glycerin acts as a humectant (a water-attracting substance). Such products physically draw water out of the skin only if used in very high concentrations. This is not to be confused with the use of 'lemon-and-glycerin' swabs. Because of the high concentration of glycerin used in these products, they can dehydrate the moist mucous membranes of the mouth. For more on this subject, see 'Use of lemon-and-glycerin swabs', this chapter, page 31.

> 'The high concentration of glycerin used in 'lemon-and-glycerin' swabs can dehydrate the moist mucous membranes of the mouth.'

Incontinence and moisture-related dermatitis
Causes

Protocols for incontinence care must include proper skin cleansing, treatment, and protection from the damaging effects of faeces, urine, and other sources of moisture (such as drainage).

Moisture-related dermatitis is due to multiple factors. These include:

- damaged skin from poor hygiene practices;
- a build-up of moisture (from urine, drainage, or sweating); and
- the effects of physical irritants (such as friction and shear forces) and chemical irritants (such as urine).

Excessive skin moisture makes the skin more permeable to irritants, and this provides an excellent medium for colonisation by pathogens. Faecal enzymes, alkaline pH, and microbial invasion (due to interaction between urine and faeces), coupled with continuing pressure or trauma to the skin, produces incontinence dermatitis. If unchecked, this eventually leads to tissue breakdown and ulcer formation.

> 'If unchecked, incontinence dermatitis eventually leads to tissue breakdown and ulcer formation.'

Barrier protectants

Barrier protectants can be of two types:

- '*dry*': transparent, water-repellent agents (such as dimethicone or other silicones); or
- '*moist*': occlusive agents (such as zinc oxide paste, petrolatum, lanolin, and wool fat derivatives).

These can be packaged in various forms—including pastes, creams, foams, and sprays (applied by hand or with applicator devices).

Products such as zinc oxide and other thick creams can repel water, but they are difficult to remove. In addition, they keep out air, as well as moisture. Cleansing the skin of these creams requires potentially damaging degrees of drag and friction. This can create further injury and trauma to skin that is already injured. The difficulties in removing these creams can lead to incomplete cleansing of the area before reapplying another application of barrier protectant cream.

Unlike 'greasy' protectants, transparent dry protectants do not interfere with the function of incontinence products. 'Greasy' protectants remain moist and the agent is transferred from the skin to the skin coverings, thus interfering with the 'wicking' action of the fibres—which are designed to draw fluids away from

> 'Greasy barrier protectants can interfere with the effectiveness of textile and disposable incontinence products.'

the skin. Because the wetness cannot be drawn into the underlying fibres, moisture spreads to other areas, thus creating larger areas of contact with the offending moisture. For these reasons, companies that produce textile and disposable incontinence products advise users to avoid use of barrier protectants because they might interfere with the effectiveness of the incontinence products.

Newer transparent barrier protectants (such as dimethicone, or combinations of dimethicone, microfine zinc oxide, and other silicone-type preparations) allow for assessment of the skin, and aid in healing by letting air circulate to tissue. Dimethicone in a concentration of 3% is especially effective if used to treat and prevent moisture-related irritation.

Barrier protectants are commonly applied to the perineum and perianal areas. However, consideration should be given to the use of these protectants in other moisture sites—such as skin folds in the obese, in the axillae and groin regions, under pendulous breasts, and behind the scrotum. Dry, breathable, and transparent barrier protectants are excellent for these areas.

Best practice in bathing
Microbiological concerns

Although bathing is an important routine for physical and emotional well-being, traditional practices of sponging commonly involve the use of one or two washcloths repeatedly plunged into a basin of increasingly soapy, 'scummy' water. This creates a 'bacteria soup', with the patient becoming dirtier (in a microbiological sense) at the end of the bath, than at the beginning (Ayliffe, Collins & Taylor 1985).

The practice of placing oils or lotions into bathwater (supposedly to 'moisturise' the skin) coats the surfaces of the basin or tub, thus creating an ideal medium for bacterial growth. It also creates a potentially hazardous situation with respect to a slick bathtub surface.

'Placing oils or lotions into bathwater coats the surfaces of the basin or tub and creates an ideal medium for bacterial growth.'

Talcum powder

Talcum powder is not advised because the 'aerosol effect' of talc can cause respiratory complications, including pneumonia and pulmonary talcosis (Nam & Gracey 1972). Patients with respiratory problems or sensitivities to perfumes and scents can also experience problems with the 'aerosol effect' of fine perfumed powders. Other talc-related concerns include: (i) an association between talc and ovarian cancer; and (ii) local skin irritation as a result of clumps of talc gathering in moisture-laden areas.

If any powder is used, it should be a non-talc product (such as cornstarch), and any powders should be used with caution in non-carpeted areas (including bathrooms) because this can lead to slick, slippery surfaces.

Basinless bathing

Proper traditional basin bathing can take up to 40 minutes. This includes obtaining and changing the water in the basin once or twice during the bath, using multiple washcloths for each part of the body (particularly genitalia and perineal areas), and then drying and applying lotions. Because there is a worldwide nursing shortage and understaffed facilities, it is not uncommon for nurses or other ancillary caregivers to take 'short cuts' in bed bathing—thus contributing to poor skin health and subsequent skin breakdown and pressure sores.

More efficient, evidence-based practice models–known as 'rinse-free basinless bathing systems'—now offer an alternative to traditional basin bathing. See Box, below.

Basinless bathing systems

Using pre-packaged soft washcloths impregnated with non-alkaline skin cleansers (to prevent dryness and thus preserve the acid mantle and natural pH of the skin), basinless bathing systems are changing the practice of bathing. These systems simultaneously cleanse and moisturise the skin, while avoiding the damaging abrasive action of washcloths.

Basinless bathing uses durable, soft, garment-like, quality washcloths (not to be confused with paper type 'hand' or 'baby' wipes). These are infused with a low-pH skin cleanser (usually < 5.5), aloe, and vitamin E to moisturise and promote skin healing. Conventional low-cost disposable or reusable washcloths can cause wound cross-contamination by fabric debris (lint) migrating into a wound or by water dripping from one part of the body to another. Disposable basinless bathing cloths are designed to be 'dripless' and lint-free. They minimise friction against sensitive skin to reduce the incidence of skin tears, particularly in older people.

The cells of the skin become hydrated in the presence of water, and moisturisers can trap this water on the skin. For this reason, moisturising agents are most effective when applied during or immediately after bathing. Basinless bathing takes advantage of this by simultaneously cleansing and moisturising the skin.

'Rinse-free' shampoo caps are also available. These products simultaneously clean and condition the hair. A new hybrid product simultaneously cleanses, moisturises, deodorises, and protects the skin.

Basinless bathing is time-efficient for nurses, yields greater satisfaction for the patient, and results in improved skin integrity.

Oral care

The importance of oral care

Poor oral hygiene and periodontal disease can be associated with diabetes, stroke, cardiovascular disease, respiratory disease, gastrointestinal problems, and adverse outcomes in pregnancy.

Best-practice models in oral hygiene consist of four essential elements:
- routine oral assessment;
- cleansing;
- debridement; and
- moisturising of the oral cavity and its structures.

Proper oral care promotes oral comfort, assists in the ability to communicate, improves nutritional status, and promotes the body's ability to fight infection; Poor or negligent oral care allows tarter to form, and this can lead to dental plaque, gingivitis, severe periodontal disease, and dysfunction.

Benefits of good oral care

Oral care:
- reduces the risk of respiratory infections;
- relieves discomfort produced by inflammation of the oral mucosa;
- improves nutritional status;
- improves speech; and
- improves outcomes for persons with wounds, stomas, or incontinence.

Adapted from Aronovitch (1997)

Dry mouth

Dry mouth can contribute to irritated gums and dental decay. The goal of good oral care is therefore to maintain mouth moisture, reduce dental plaque, and decrease mouth bacteria to prevent colonisation of dental plaque.

Many medications play a role in the production of dry mouth, especially some antihypertensives and antibiotics. For those with significantly reduced saliva production, a saliva substitute or *mucoadhesive gel* can be used to produce or replace moisture. These maintain mouth moistness over long periods of time by leaving a coating on the mucosa and oral structures to maintain oral moistness and promote saliva. Mouth pain can also be reduced using these gels because they adhere to irritated tissue, thus decreasing airflow to the area.

Plaque

Plaque is one of the leading factors in gum disease. Problems start with the formation of tartar, which provides a rough surface on which bacterial dental plaque can form. It is imperative that diligent cleaning be undertaken of the teeth, false teeth, and the insides of the cheek and mouth to reduce dental plaque. Good oral hygiene is essential, regardless of a person's age and the number of natural teeth that the person has.

'Good oral hygiene is essential, regardless of a peron's age and the number of natural teeth that the person has.'

Debridement

Mechanical and chemical debridement of the oral mucosa and teeth reduces dental plaque and mouth bacteria, and also stimulates the production of saliva. The avoidance or removal of dental plaque is a significant factor in preventing mouth infections.

'Meticulous oral care must be part of any infection-control policy.'

This is therefore an important nursing responsibility. Poor oral hygiene and periodontal disease leads to colonisation of the mouth with bacteria, and subsequent microaspiration can lead to respiratory infections. Persons at risk include the elderly, those with chronic aspiration problems, those receiving tube feedings, and those intubated or with a tracheostomy. Meticulous oral care must be part of any infection-control policy.

In attempting to maintain cleanliness, prevent infection, moisturise the oral cavity, maintain mucosal integrity, and promote healing, oral care agents should (Beck & Yasko 1993):

▶ be mechanically and chemically atraumatic;
▶ be non-decalcifying and non-toxic;
▶ not interfere with saliva;

▶ have acceptable odour and taste;
▶ provide mechanical or chemical action to remove debris; and
▶ provide moistening and lubricating action.

Undesirable practices

Unfortunately, traditional oral care has been fragmented and creative. The following practices are not based on good evidence, and should therefore be discouraged.

▶ use of inappropriate instruments and swabs;
▶ use of citric juices or 'home-made' brews to cleanse the mouth; and
▶ use of lemon-and-glycerin swabs.
   Each of these is discussed below.

Use of inappropriate instruments and swabs

For residents unable to perform self-care with a toothbrush, nurses have used lemon-and-glycerin swabs, cotton-tip swabs (often dipped in sodium bicarbonate or dentifrice), gauze sponges wrapped on forceps, tongue depressors, and gauze wrapped around fingers. Some caregivers have used hard-edged implements to pry open (or prop open) the mouth.

These practices are potentially dangerous because cotton applicators leave behind small fibres that residents can swallow or inhale. Fibres can become trapped in the oral cavity causing bacterial seeding. Wood or hard-edged implements can cause wounds to the oral cavity. In addition, the fingers of caregivers can be bitten.

Use of citric juices or 'home-made' brews to cleanse the mouth

Carbonated drinks and commercially prepared fruit juices are acidic and can further demineralise the teeth. Alcohol-based mouthwashes can act as oral irritants, can dry out the oral mucosa, and have been linked with the occurrence of oral cancer (Beck & Yasko 2001).

Use of lemon-and-glycerin swabs

Despite their popularity, these swabs have no mechanical or cleansing value, and there is no evidence to support their continued use. They are acidic, and this can damage teeth and promote mouth infections (Passos & Brand 1966). In addition, glycerin absorbs water, thus drying out oral tissues.

Despite warnings in the literature about the effects of these swabs (Passos & Brand 1966), many nurses continue to use them. Apart from the effects of the lemon and glycerine in these products, cotton swabs are not designed for oral hygiene, offer no mechanical debridement, and should never be used as part of routine oral care.

Evidence-based oral care

Toothbrushes and alternatives

Best practice in oral cleansing is achieved by using an ultra-soft toothbrush with toothpaste for at least two minutes. False teeth also require diligent cleansing, and should not merely be dipped or soaked in water.

Toothbrushes that are too hard can injure the oral tissues. Electric toothbrushes are gaining popularity with older persons because they are easier to use and provide improved cleansing action. However, for people with dementia or other conditions causing cognitive impairment, the vibrations and noise can be disturbing. 'Twin-headed' toothbrushes are an alternative, and these can simultaneously cleanse the front and back surfaces of the teeth.

For some people, neither electric toothbrushes nor manual toothbrushes are appropriate. These include people who are 'mouth phobic', those who bleed easily, those who have oral trauma, those who are unconscious, or those who are otherwise severely incapacitated. For these people, alternatives to toothbrushes are required. Dense foam-tipped oral swabs (commonly referred to as 'toothettes') containing deep grooves or ridges can mimic the actions of a toothbrush. These debride and clean the surface of the teeth (and in between the teeth), as well as cleaning the oral mucosa and hard palate. As with a toothbrush, a dentifrice compound (toothpaste or other agent) is used in conjunction with these oral foam swabs.

Mouth props

For people who are unable to cooperate with oral care, the traditional hard implements used to pry open or prop open the mouth should not be used. These can be replaced with a 'bite block' or 'mouth prop' made out of dense dental foam. This cannot be bitten off, and does not injure the teeth, mouth, or gums. The use of this foam is particularly appropriate in providing oral care for people with dementia, strokes, or spasticity problems because it adds a measure of safety for both resident and caregiver.

'A 'bite block' or 'mouth prop' made of dense dental foam adds a measure of safety for both resident and caregiver.'

Cleansing agents

A combination of sodium bicarbonate (baking soda) and a 1.5% hydrogen peroxide solution is superior to the cleansing action of dentifrice. Hydrogen peroxide is an effective agent that mechanically cleanses by working in conjunction with saliva to 'froth and bubble', thus loosening degenerated tissue, debris, and mucus. The combination of hydrogen peroxide and baking soda breaks down secretions, provides excellent debridement, and offers antimicrobial action for the mucosa and teeth (Beck & Yasko 1993). Care should be taken that it is not swallowed.

Other cleansing procedures use sodium bicarbonate in combination with an antiseptic oral rinse containing enzymes to aid the debriding action of saliva. The use of these products is not to be confused with traditional antiseptic mouth rinses (such as thymol and chlorhexidine), which offer no mechanical debriding or cleansing properties.

Chlorhexidine mouthwash is often misused as part of routine oral care. It is not intended for long-term use and is not a replacement for proper oral cleansing and debridement. Side-effects include staining of the teeth, alterations in taste, parotitis, calculus formation, and increased tartar and plaque formation. Chlorhexidine should be used in conjunction with effective oral care, not in place of it. It should be used after oral hygiene, and should not be swallowed. The mouth should not be rinsed with water or mouthwash.

> 'Chlorhexidine mouthwash is not a replacement for proper oral cleansing and debridement.'

Conclusion

Older people's nurses should become proactive in developing evidence-based skin and oral care. Tradition should give way to new technology and advances, even if they challenge long-held beliefs.

Prevention is the key to reducing infections, and this starts with changing the most basic of practices in oral and skin hygiene. Applying science and technology to hygiene practices ensures resident comfort, effective skin care, and oral health, and elevates the most fundamental of nursing procedures to newer evolving standards.

Chapter 4

Pressure Ulcers and Leg Ulcers

Sue Templeton

Introduction

Wound management involves much more than treating the wound; wound management involves caring for *the person* with a wound. Each person with a wound should be treated in an holistic manner that includes the physical, psychological, emotional, and social effects of the wound on that person.

Wound management is a constantly evolving area of health care, and new treatments are being developed and released every year. To deliver optimal wound management, nurses must continually update their knowledge and skills, and the use of current, evidence-based protocols and practices is necessary for sound wound-management practice in care of older people.

Wound management

Principles

In assessing and treating any wound, sound wound-management principles should always be followed. The principles of wound management are (Fergusson & McLellan 1997):

▶ determine the cause of the wound;

▶ identify factors that might impair healing;

▶ control or eliminate factors that might impair healing;

▶ determine long-term and short-term objectives;

▶ implement an appropriate wound-management regimen;

▶ evaluate, reassess, and revise the management regimen frequently; and

▶ plan for maintenance of healed tissue.

Assessment

Before selecting a dressing and other therapies with a view to providing ideal conditions at the wound site to facilitate healing, comprehensive and systematic assessment is required. Such an assessment helps to identify the cause of the wound (MacLellan & Rice 1995), and the identification of factors that might impair healing or prevent a wound responding to dressings alone (Holt et al. 1992; Doughty 1992). For example, if a person has had radiotherapy to an area, this might have damaged the tissues, thus making would healing difficult in this area.

Corticosteroid medication also impairs wound healing. If people are receiving such treatment for rheumatoid arthritis or other conditions requiring ongoing steroid therapy, it is often not desirable to cease their corticosteroid medication. In these and similar cases, healing can be an unrealistic objective.

Bacterial load at the wound site might also inhibit healing. The term 'bacterial load' refers to the number of bacteria in a wound. A wound with a high bacterial load might not exhibit obvious signs of infection (such as purulent exudate and erythema), but a high bacterial load can nevertheless impair or prevent healing (Falanga 2001). Many chronic wounds have such a high bacterial load, and treatment to reduce this can be undertaken through the use of dressings containing cadexomer iodine or ionised silver (Sundberg & Meller 1997; Sibbald et al. 2001).

Figure 4.1 (page 37) illustrates these and other factors that can impair wound healing.

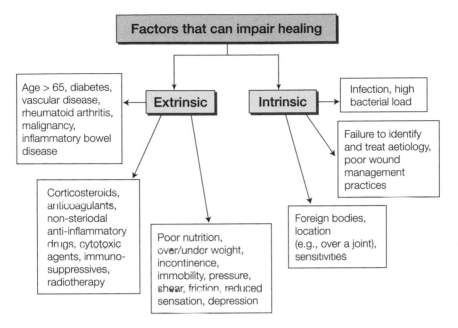

Figure 4.1 Factors that can impair healing
Author's creation

A management regimen

An evidence-based management regimen should be implemented, and realistic and achievable objectives, both long term and short term, should be decided. These will provide guidance for the treatment plan and facilitate ongoing assessment of that plan.

Dressings form only one component of this. A management regimen should also include other interventions—such as nutritional and/or vitamin supplementation, use of pressure-reducing devices, skin care, compression therapy, limb elevation, footwear assessment, improved control of diabetes, medication review, increased exercise, and cessation of smoking.

In choosing dressings, certain criteria should be kept in mind. The dressing should (Doughty 1992):

▶ keep the wound environment moist (but not wet);
▶ debride any slough (or necrotic tissue);
▶ ensure that any cavities or dead spaces are filled (but not tightly packed);
▶ keep the wound temperature at 37 degrees Celsius;
▶ not adhere to the wound, or leak within 24 hours;
▶ protect the surrounding skin from trauma (caused by tapes or dressings, body fluids, or wound exudate);

- not support bacterial growth; and
- be cost-effective

Nurses should understand the function of each dressing, how to apply it appropriately, and the expected outcome of its use.

Dressings should be chosen according to the level of wound exudate. The ideal wound environment is moist, but not wet (Carville 2001). A moist wound environment provides the optimal conditions for wound healing to occur. Moist wound healing occurs faster than dry wound healing. Epidermal cells will migrate across only a moist surface (Dealey 1994).

Figure 4.2 (page 39) provides a guide to choosing dressings with a view to promoting a moist wound-healing environment.

There are numerous dressings available, and no single dressing is suitable for all wounds (Doughty 1992). In addition, a single dressing is often not suitable for the duration of a wound. A management regimen that has positive outcomes for one person might not be suitable for another. Each person and his or her wound must be assessed on an individual basis, and a management regimen must be tailored to that person's specific characteristics.

> 'Each person and wound must be assessed on an individual basis.'

Pressure ulcers
Aetiology

Pressure ulcers result from tissue damage caused by unrelieved, focal pressure (Dealey 1994). When body tissues are compressed against a hard surface (such as a bony prominence), capillaries are closed off, and the consequent reduction in blood flow causes hypoxia in the area. If the pressure is not relieved, the capillaries rupture and leak, resulting in non-blanching erythema (Bryant et al. 1992). Non-blanching erythema is an ominous sign of tissue damage. Ongoing, unrelieved pressure results in a cycle of inflammation, hypoxia, oedema, ischaemia, and necrosis that extends the area of tissue damage (Carville 2001; Bryant et al. 1992). Eventually, tissue breakdown occurs. Because muscle and fat are more susceptible to the effects of pressure than is skin, damage to the internal tissues can be more extensive than what is apparent on the skin (Maklebust & Sieggreen 2001).

An individual's susceptibility to pressure-related tissue damage varies. It is dependent on (AWMA 2001):

- the intensity and duration of pressure; and
- the tolerance of the tissues to pressure.

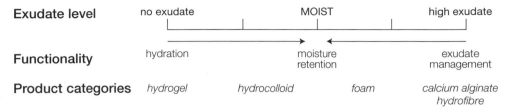

Exudate level	no exudate		MOIST		high exudate

Functionality	hydration		moisture retention		exudate management

| Product categories | hydrogel | hydrocolloid | | foam | calcium alginate hydrofibre |

Figure 4.2 Choosing dressings to promote a moist environment

Author's creation

Prevention

Strategies for prevention of pressure-related damage

Effective skin care is vital to the prevention of pressure ulcers. When assisting older people in their care with daily hygiene, nurses have an excellent opportunity to inspect skin condition carefully. At this time it is easy to observe skin turgor, moisture level, colour, and texture. Ensuring that wounds and skin conditions are not overlooked does require some training, and a program of training in skin assessment is recommended for all nurses working with older persons. With sound assessment skills, potential pressure areas can be identified early and action taken to avoid skin breakdown.

Risk assessment

It is vital to determine which individuals are at risk of developing pressure ulcers. The factors that place an individual at greater risk of developing a pressure ulcer have been incorporated into various risk-assessment scales. These scales rate various factors that can contribute to pressure ulcer development and express this rating as a numerical score (Newman & Lim 2001). The most important factors are:

▶ *immobility:* the inability to change position voluntarily; and
▶ *decreased sensory perception:* a reduced ability to sense discomfort and pain.

Other factors that can contribute to pressure-related damage include (AMWA 2001):

▶ shear and/or friction;
▶ moisture, especially from faecal or urinary incontinence;
▶ age greater than 65 years;
▶ poor nutrition; and
▶ poor circulation.

The most commonly used risk-assessment scales are the Norton scale (1989), the Waterlow scale (1985), and the Braden scale (1987). An effective scale should indicate whether an individual is at low, moderate, high, or very high risk of developing pressure ulcers. Pressure ulcer risk-assessment scales have received some criticism for over-predicting risk and for a lack of valid research studies to support their use (Banks 1998). However, the use of risk-assessment tools has many benefits—including effective use of resources, facilitation of auditing, improvement in standards, minimisation of risk, and protection against litigation (Banks 1998).

Prevention of pressure ulcers

In addition to the systematic, regular assessment of risk, it is vital to ensure that evidence-based strategies are used that translate the risk score into practical nursing interventions (Maklebust & Sieggreen 2001). After all, practical interventions, not the completion of a risk-assessment score, prevent the development of a pressure ulcer. The introduction of any pressure ulcer risk-assessment scale must be undertaken in association with a comprehensive education strategy and implementation plan to ensure that effective use is made of the information gained from using the scale. Table 4.1 (below) presents some useful strategies and the rationale for each.

Table 4.1 Strategies and rationales in wound management

Strategy	Rationale
Control of excess moisture (incontinence, perspiration, wound exudate)	Excess moisture can cause maceration of the skin
Avoid dry skin	Dry skin can crack
	A cleanser with a pH close to that of the skin should be used (pH 4.0–6.8)
Good nutritional status and fluid balance	Supplementation needs to be considered (vitamins, high-energy and high-protein drinks, enteral feeding)
Repositioning of an immobile person frequently	Frequency of repositioning is based on frequent skin inspection and skin's tolerance to pressure
	Pillows or foam should be used to reduce pressure between bony prominences

(Continued)

Table 4.1 Strategies and rationales in wound management (*Continued*)

Strategy	Rationale
Avoid use of doughnut-shaped devices	These are not effective
Avoid massaging of bony prominences	This can cause deep tissue damage
Avoid raising the bed head higher than 30 degrees	A bed head raised more than 30 degrees results in increased shear forces because the person slides down the bed
Raise the foot end of the bed slightly	This can help prevent sliding down the bed by providing counter-traction.
Avoid placing the knees or feet higher than the hips when a person is sitting	If knees or feet are higher than the hips, the ischial tuberosities are made more prominent, thus increasing pressure to the buttocks
Use lifting aids when moving immobile persons	This reduces friction and reduces the risk of personal injury
Use a pressure-reducing or pressure-relieving device suitable for the assessed level of risk	These devices distribute pressure over a greater surface area or relieve pressure from the body

Author's creation adapted from JBI (1997); AWMA (2001)

Pressure-reducing and pressure-relieving devices

There are many pressure-reducing and pressure-relieving devices on the market. The choice of which device to use should be linked to the score obtained from a risk-assessment scale (see Figure 4.3, below).

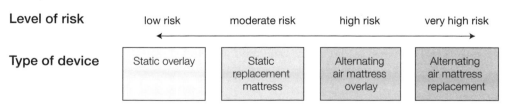

Figure 4.3 Choosing pressure-reducing and pressure-relieving devices

Author's creation adapted from Australian Wound Management Association (2001)

Definitions

Overlay: a device that is laid over an existing mattress

Mattress replacement: a device that replaces the existing mattress.

Static device: a device that does not have any independent movement, but relies on body weight to change its shape; usually these devices do not require electricity.

Dynamic device: a device that alters its shape according to a predetermined cycle. These devices usually require electricity to operate a pump.

Generally, a thicker mattress provides more effective pressure relief or reduction. For example, a shallow air-mattress overlay is not recommended for a person who is at very high risk because it will not provide adequate pressure reduction over bony prominences (McLeod 1997). For a person at very high risk, a mattress-replacement system that has cells at least 190 mm thick is recommended (McLeod 1997).

When selecting a pressure-reducing or pressure-relieving device, it is important to have knowledge of the person's requirements and the specific

Table 4.2 Stage classification of pressure ulcers

Stage	Description
Stage I	Non-blanchable erythema of intact skin. In persons with lighter skin this can appear as a persistent reddened patch. In persons with darker skin this can appear as a red, blue, or purple coloured area.
Stage II	A partial thickness wound that involves loss of the epidermis and/or dermis. The wound is superficial and can appear as an abrasion or shallow crater.
Stage III	A full-thickness wound that extends into the subcutaneous fat layer, but does not involve the underlying fascia. The wound can be deep; undermining of surrounding tissues can be present.
Stage IV	A full-thickness wound that extends through the fascia. The wound can involve damage or necrosis of muscle and deeper structures such as bone, joint capsule, and tendon. Extensive undermining and sinus tracts can be present. **Note:** A pressure ulcer cannot be adequately staged in the presence of necrotic tissue or a blister.

Author's creation adapted from AWMA (2001); Maklebust & Sieggreen (2001)

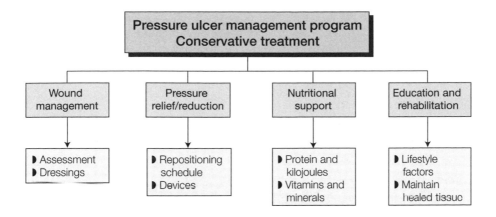

Figure 4.4 Conservative treatment of pressure ulcers
Author's creation

characteristics of the device to ensure that it will meet the person's needs (Hopkins, Gooch & Danks 1998). An understanding of how to operate and maintain the device is also necessary. It is important that nurses recognise that a mattress must prevent capillaries from reaching 'closing pressure' if pressure is to be reduced or relieved adequately.

Treatment

Conservative treatment

A pressure ulcer treatment program involves a multi-faceted approach, with numerous, related factors needing to be considered if a pressure ulcer is to be healed and its recurrence prevented.

Conservative treatment is the main form of management, particularly for older persons. Reconstructive surgery is the last resort in the treatment of pressure ulcers. See Figure 4.4, (above) for a summary of conservative measures in treatment of pressure ulcers.

Staging of pressure ulcers

A four-stage classification system for pressure ulcers is widely accepted (see Table 4.2, page 42). This system is based on the depth of the wound and the structures involved.

A pressure ulcer staging system is only one component of the assessment of a person with a pressure ulcer. A comprehensive, systematic assessment is vital to ensure that the most effective treatment program is implemented.

Wound management

A thorough assessment of the wound must be undertaken to determine the true extent of the wound. The following factors should be considered in selecting a wound-management program.

Debridement

Necrotic and sloughy tissue should be removed from the wound. The presence of necrosis and slough increases the risk of infection, prevents proper assessment, and can obscure abscesses or fluid collections (Carville 2001; Maklebust & Sieggreen 2001).

Sharp debridement uses sterile scalpels, scissors, or lasers to remove necrosis or slough quickly and effectively. Sharp debridement should be performed only by a surgeon or a registered nurse who is clinically competent in this procedure (Carville 2001).

Autolytic debridement uses dressings to provide a moist wound environment to assist in the breakdown of necrotic tissue (Maklebust & Sieggreen 2001). This is the preferred method because it is simple, effective, and selective.

Dressings

Dressings should be chosen according to the guidelines outlined at the beginning of this chapter. It should be remembered that no single dressing is suitable for every person and that no single dressing is suitable for the life of a wound.

> 'No single dressing is suitable for every person and no single dressing is suitable for the life of a wound.

In managing pressure ulcers, the following considerations are of particular importance in relation to dressings:

- ▶ when filling a large cavity or sinus, choose dressings that will not lose their form when moist;
- ▶ whenever possible, use only one piece of dressing in a wound, particularly if undermining or sinuses are present; dressings or dressing residue left in the wound can impair healing and increase the risk of infection.

Evaluation of progress

A stage III or IV pressure ulcer healing by secondary intention can take many months to heal. Frequent evaluation and documentation of wound dimensions and characteristics should be undertaken by a nurse at least weekly to ensure healing is progressing (Maklebust & Sieggreen 2001).

Lack of progress or deterioration of a pressure wound can indicate infection, inadequate pressure reduction, poor fluid and nutritional status, and/or inappropriate dressing choices. Management should involve identification and treatment of the contributing factors.

A multidisciplinary team approach ensures the best possible outcome for people with pressure ulcers. This might involve a nurse, a wound specialist, a general practitioner, a specialist medical practitioner, a dietitian, a physiotherapist, an occupational therapist, and others.

Leg ulcers

A leg ulcer can be defined as a wound below the knee that does not heal in six weeks (Scully 1999). The term 'leg ulcer', on its own, is not a diagnosis (Cullum & Roe 1998). Any non-healing wound on the lower limb should be investigated to determine *why* it is not healing.

The main cause of leg ulcers is circulatory insufficiency (Morison et al. 1997). Leg ulcers can occur spontaneously or develop following minor trauma. Other causes of leg ulcers that should be excluded include chronic infections, malignancy, and haematological conditions (Thursby 1993).

Venous leg ulcers

Venous insufficiency of the deep veins accounts for the majority of leg ulcers (Cullum & Roe 1998). As valves in the veins fail, increased pressure occurs within the deep vein system. This pressure is transmitted, leading to increased pressure in the superficial venous system (Morison et al. 1997). This increased pressure can result in a venous ulcer.

Signs that can indicate venous ulcers include (Carville 2001):

▶ an ulcer in the 'gaiter' region of the leg (the lower one-third of the leg, including the ankles);
▶ pulses usually present (although it can be difficult to palpate the foot pulses in the presence of oedema);
▶ a shallow ulcer with poorly defined margins;
▶ slow ulcer progression;
▶ reports of discomfort (rather than severe pain);
▶ discomfort relieved on elevation of the limb;
▶ ulcer base containing granulation tissue; and
▶ history of deep vein thrombosis (DVT), pulmonary embolus (PE), trauma or surgery to the leg, and/or obesity.

Table 4.3 Presentation and pathophysiology of venous leg ulcers

Clinical presentation	Pathophysiology
Varicose veins	High pressures in the superficial venous system due to valve failure
Oedema	Capillaries 'leak' water and plasma proteins into the tissues
Brown staining of the skin	As capillaries become further damaged they 'leak' red blood cells into the tissues
Eczema	Irritation of the skin due to breakdown of haemoglobin and accumulation of toxins
Hardness (fibrosis) of gaiter area (inverted champagne bottle leg)	Effects of chronic fat necrosis, inflammation, induration, and scarring resulting from the above pathophysiologies

Author's creation adapted from Cullum & Roe (1998); Vowden (1998)

A diagnosis of a venous leg ulcer can be made only after a comprehensive and systematic assessment of the person's medical conditions and a clinical assessment of the limb and wound.

Graduated compression bandaging has been demonstrated to be the most effective therapy for the treatment of venous leg ulcers (Fletcher, Cullum & Sheldon 1997: Cullum et al. 1998). Graduated compression therapy acts by providing a firm casing around the leg, which assists in forcing fluid from the leg, which assists in forcing fluid from the tissues back into the vascular and lymphatic systems (Thomas 1996). A compression level of 35–40 mm Hg at the ankle has been reported to be optimal, reducing to approximately 20 mm Hg at the knee (Morison et al. 1997). This can be attained through the use of 4-layer compression bandaging, short stretch compression bandaging, or long stretch compression bandaging.

The use of a zinc paste bandage under compression bandaging can be an effective treatment for dermatitis or venous eczema (Carville 2001). To obtain the best results, an appropriate bandage should be selected and correctly applied by a trained nurse (Nelson 1996). However, graduated compression therapy corrects only the symptoms of venous insufficiency; it does not cure the valvular incompetence.

Once venous leg ulcers have been healed, compression stockings of

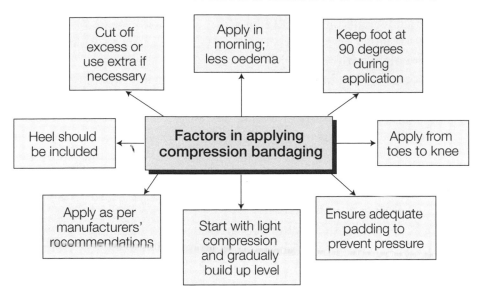

Figure 4.5 Factors in applying compression bandaging
Author's creation

approximately 20–25 mm Hg should be worn during the day to prevent recurrence of ulceration (Morison et al. 1997).

Dressings can be applied under compression therapy and should be selected according to the exudate level and characteristics of the wound.

Arterial leg ulcers

Arterial insufficiency is the next most common cause of leg ulcers after venous causes. This is usually due to the effects of atherosclerosis and calcification of the arteries. Arterial leg ulcers result from a lack of arterial blood supply, leading to tissue ischaemia and necrosis (Morison et al. 1997).

Clinical signs that indicate an arterial ulcer include the following (Carville 2001; Dealey 1994):

▶ absence of oedema;
▶ ulcer on the malleolus, foot, or toes;
▶ pulses usually weak or absent;
▶ deep ulcer with a 'punched-out' appearance;
▶ rapid progress;
▶ often associated with severe pain that might require narcotic analgesia;
▶ pain reported to be worse at night or on elevation of the limb;
▶ ulcer base often contains sloughy and/or necrotic tissue;

> thickened toenails, absence of hair, shiny skin; and
> history of cardiac disease, hypertension, cerebrovascular accident, myocardial infarction, diabetes, and/or smoking.

A person with the clinical signs of arterial ulceration should be referred to a vascular surgeon for further assessment and treatment (Carville 2001). Nursing objectives include the control of risk factors (if possible), prevention of infection, and sound wound-management practices (Morison et al. 1997). Ulcers due to severe arterial disease are very unlikely to heal with dressings alone (Smith 2002). Compression bandaging should not be used on persons with arterial disease because this can restrict the circulation and can cause severe tissue damage (Cullum & Roe 1998).

Surgical options for the treatment of arterial ulcers aim to improve the arterial supply. Interventions include chemical or surgical sympathectomy, angioplasty, vascular bypass surgery, and amputation (Carville 2001).

Mixed vessel ulcers

Some people present with clinical signs that suggest that their ulcers are due to a combination of venous and arterial disease. The likelihood of these ulcers healing is dependent on the degree of arterial disease.

Light compression bandaging might be possible if the arterial disease is not severe (Smith 2002). A thorough assessment and an individualised treatment plan is required to manage this challenging problem.

Ulcers related to diabetes

Lower-limb ulcers can also be attributed to the complications of diabetes. This can be the result of a number of conditions—including arterial disease, venous disease, and autonomic, sensory, and motor neuropathy (Morison et al. 1997).

Venous and arterial disease, if present, should be treated as outlined above. Minimisation of the effects of neuropathy is best achieved by referral to a podiatrist to ensure appropriate footwear, pressure offloading, and treatment of foot problems (Carville 2001).

Conclusion

Wound management in older people can present many challenges. A thorough assessment should be undertaken of the person, taking into consideration all medical, surgical, social, and psychological factors. Because ageing produces a number of physiological changes that can affect healing, nursing an older person with a wound can often be frustrating. Whatever the aetiology and potential for healing, all nurses have a responsibility to ensure that interventions ensure the best quality of life for the person with a wound.

Sound, evidence-based knowledge, the ability to communicate effectively with others, and the involvement of patients to the best of their ability will all assist a nurse in achieving a sense of professional and personal satisfaction in caring for an older person with a wound.

'Nurses have a responsibility to ensure that interventions ensure the best quality of life for the person with a wound.'

Chapter 5

Foot Care

Hylton Menz

Introduction

Foot problems are a common accompaniment of advancing age, and are associated with impaired mobility, limited independence, and diminished quality of life. Despite the significant impact that foot problems have on the lives of older people, these problems can easily be overlooked by medical and nursing staff. Because older people themselves often consider foot pain to be an unavoidable consequence of ageing (Williamson, Stokoe & Gray 1964), they might not report foot problems when providing their medical history. In addition, many nurses do not consider themselves to be sufficiently knowledgeable about foot problems to initiate preventative treatment (Pierson 1991; Love 1995). Many older people thus needlessly endure pain and disability—despite the fact that many foot ailments can be prevented or managed with conservative interventions.

'Many older people needlessly endure pain and disability.'

Prevalence of foot problems

Foot problems are common in older people. However, there is a lack of reliable data on the prevalence of foot problems in older people, and the studies that have been conducted have reported quite disparate findings. There are two reasons for this: (i) uncertainty regarding the definition of a 'foot problem'; and (ii) different populations having been studied.

In *defining* what actually constitutes a 'foot problem', some studies have relied on clinicians to assess and document observed foot problems, whereas others have relied upon subjective reports by older people themselves. Both approaches have their limitations—clinicians might detect foot conditions that have little effect on the older person's lifestyle, whereas older people might attribute their pain or decreased mobility to other factors (when, in fact, their foot conditions might be the primary cause).

With respect to the *population* being assessed, studies conducted in hospitals or clinical settings have reported very high rates of foot problems—up to 80% of older people (Hung Ho & Leung 1985; Ebrahim, Sainsbury, & Watson 1981; Crawford et al. 1995). In contrast, studies in the wider community have reported much lower rates of foot problems—generally in the range of 30–40% (Greenberg 1994).

Irrespective of the method of ascertaining foot problems and the population being assessed, there is a general consensus that older women are three times more likely to suffer from foot problems than men—which has been attributed to ill-fitting footwear (Gorecki 1978; Frey et al. 1993).

The prevalence of foot problems certainly increases with age. However, in the very old, many foot problems are less significant because these people are more likely to have reduced mobility or be confined to bed.

The most common foot problems in older people are chronic in nature and reflect the long-term physiological changes that occur to the sensory, muscular, articular, neurological, and vascular systems. By far the most common problems are hyperkeratotic lesions (corns and calluses), followed closely by nail disorders and structural deformities such as hallux valgus (bunions) and lesser-toe deformities (hammer toes and claw toes). Many

'Older women are three times more likely to suffer from foot problems—due to ill-fitting footwear.'

functional foot disorders (for example, those caused by impaired lower limb mechanics when walking) are also common in older people—but these are often not adequately evaluated, diagnosed, or managed.

Consequences of foot problems

The main reason for older people seeking treatment for foot problems is disabling pain. However, even in the absence of obvious foot discomfort, foot problems can contribute to impaired physical functioning in the activities of daily living—such as housework, gardening, shopping, cooking, and cleaning. Older people with foot problems walk more slowly and have more problems with balance (Menz & Lord 2001)—which increases the risk of accidental falls.

'The main reason for older people seeking treatment for foot problems is disabling pain.'

For people with diabetes mellitus, apparently trivial foot conditions take on even greater significance. An untreated ingrown toenail or corn can lead to ulceration, infection, and even amputation. Untreated calluses are a common precursor to plantar ulcers (Murray et al. 1996), and the presence of skin fissures or ingrown toenails can double the risk of lower limb amputation (Flores-Rivera 1998).

Older people's nurses can have a significant effect on the quality of life of those in their care by detecting these problems at an early stage, and instituting appropriate management.

'Nurses can have a significant effect on the quality of life of those in their care.'

The effects of ageing

As with many conditions in older people, it is often difficult to differentiate between foot conditions caused by normal ageing and those caused by disease.

As people become older, the skin on the foot becomes drier and the epidermis is significantly thinner and less resilient—leading to an increased risk of fissuring. In addition, ageing causes impaired tactile sensitivity and a diminished awareness of foot position. There is also a flattening of the dermo–epidermal junction with age, and this decreases the mechanical resistance of the skin to shearing forces.

Circulatory problems increase with ageing. Reduced peripheral blood supply leads to impaired healing and increased prevalence of arterial ulceration. Impaired venous return can produce ankle oedema, telangiectasia, varicose veins, and ulceration (especially in the medial ankle region). Chilblains are also common in older people with impaired peripheral circulation. These itchy (and often painful) lesions on the toes are caused by an abnormal vascular reaction to localised warming of the tissues.

The flexibility of the many joints in the foot decreases with age. In particular, ankle joint movements are markedly decreased, and this makes the foot less able to absorb the 'shock' experienced when walking. Restricted range of motion in the foot also makes it more difficult for older people to maintain balance when walking on irregular terrain—thus contributing to falls. Ligaments become stiffer and less resilient with advancing age, and this is of particular importance to the structure and function of the foot. The phrase 'fallen arches' describes the effect of a weakening of the plantar calcaneo–navicular ligament—which is partly responsible for maintaining the medial arch of the foot. The weakening of this ligament allows gravity to lower the arch. Similarly, many older people notice that their feet 'spread' with age. This is due to the reduced resilience of the transverse metatarsal ligaments that are responsible for holding the metatarsal bones of the foot in alignment. The combined effect of reduced ligament resilience and altered muscle function can also contribute to common structural foot deformities in older people—such as hallux valgus ('bunions') and lesser-toe deformity ('hammer toes' and 'claw toes').

Management of common foot problems

Nurses are often in the best position to detect foot problems. In addition, if there are no podiatry services available, nurses are sometimes called upon to attend to basic foot needs—such as toenail reduction and management of superficial skin problems.

The following categories of foot problems are discussed below:
▶ nail disorders;
▶ skin disorders;
▶ structural foot problems; and
▶ functional foot problems.

Nail disorders

Nail disorders are common among older people. Although these are often considered to be trivial conditions, nail disorders can be extremely painful and can lead to quite serious secondary infection (especially in immuno-compromised persons).

The nail conditions affecting older people are:
▶ onychauxis;
▶ onychocryptosis;

▶ onychomycosis; and
▶ other nail conditions.

Onychauxis

Onychauxis is the name given to *abnormal thickening of the nail*. This can result from a range of causes—including injury, trauma from ill-fitting shoes, infection, peripheral vascular disease, diabetes, and nutritional deficiency. A more severe form of the condition—often called *onychogryphosis* or 'ram's horn nail'—results from long-term neglect and is characterised by thickening in conjunction with pronounced curvature. Onychauxis and onychogryphosis are often accompanied by *onychophosis*—the formation of callus in the nail grooves.

In some cases of onychauxis, pressure from bedclothes or tight hosiery can lead to quite severe pain. If left untreated, a subungual haematoma (blood blister under the nail) can form, creating a potential site for infection.

Regular basic foot hygiene, including filing of nails, can prevent excessive build-up of thickened nail. However, more severe cases require treatment by a podiatrist using a special drill to reduce the thickness of the nail.

Onychocryptosis

The term *onychocryptosis* refers to 'ingrown' toenails. A spicule of nail penetrates the skin, leading to inflammation, pain, and increased risk of secondary infection. People with abnormally curved nails or overriding toes are more likely to develop onychocryptosis. However, in many cases, the condition is simply caused by inappropriate nail cutting and/or ill-fitting footwear. Toenails should be cut straight across, and shoes should have sufficient room in the toe-box to prevent constriction.

Some cases can be successfully managed by applying topical antiseptics and allowing the nail to grow out normally, but recurrent cases can require a minor surgical procedure performed by a podiatrist. This involves removing the offending portion of nail under local anaesthetic, and applying a caustic solution to destroy some of the cells that produce the nail plate. This makes the nail narrower and prevents regrowth. Although this technique takes slightly longer to heal than incisional surgery, it is associated with a significantly lower rate of recurrence and is therefore the treatment of choice (Rounding & Hulm 2000).

Onychomycosis

The term *onychomycosis* refers to fungal nail infection—usually caused by dermatophyte, saprophyte, and yeast organisms. Fungal infection of the nail is extremely common in older people, and results in yellow-brown discoloration, thickening, crumbling, and offensive odour.

Although it is often considered a trivial complaint, onychomycosis is not merely a cosmetic problem. The condition produces adverse psychosocial and physical effects that can diminish quality of life, and fungal nail infection increases the risk of ingrown toenails—which often cause quite severe pain and secondary infection.

Conscientious management of foot hygiene, including careful washing and drying of the feet, can prevent many fungal nail infections. Shoes, socks, or hosiery should be changed daily to prevent moisture build-up.

Once the condition has developed, it can take some time to achieve a complete cure. A range of treatments is used to treat the condition. However, the best treatment is terbinafine (Lamisil)—an oral medication that has been shown to cure the condition in 3–6 months with minimal side effects (Evans & Sigurgeirsson 1999). If oral medication is contraindicated, topical treatments (such as azoles, tolnaftate, or undecenoic acid preparations) can be used. However, these take much longer, require careful compliance, and have significantly lower cure rates (Hart et al. 1999).

'Conscientious management of foot hygiene can prevent many fungal nail infections.'

Other nail problems

Other nail conditions that can present in older persons include *paronychia* (inflammation of the surrounding tissue of the nail), *onycholysis* (separation of the nail plate, often associated with trauma), and *onychomalacia* (excessively soft nails).

Many nail changes are indicative of underlying systemic conditions. For example, *leukonychia* (white nails) can indicate underlying liver disease, and *hippocratic nails* (clubbed nails) are associated with a range of lung diseases, cardiovascular diseases, and thyroid disease. Nurses should be alert to the possibility that nail changes might indicate a more serious underlying disease. Any recent changes in the appearance of an older person's nails should be documented and referred to a physician or podiatrist for further evaluation.

'Any recent changes in the appearance of an older person's nails should be documented and referred for further evaluation.'

Skin disorders

Hyperkeratosis (epidermal thickening) is a normal physiological response to friction, and acts as a protective mechanism to prevent damage to deeper tissues. The foot is a common site for hyperkeratosis to develop because the skin on the foot is subject to friction from footwear and weight-bearing. The resultant focal thickening can become extremely painful, can increase pressure on the underlying dermis, and can lead to ulceration.

There are two types of hyperkeratosis:

▶ *calluses*—which usually develop on the plantar surface of the foot and appear as a diffuse thickening; and

▶ *corns*—which are more common on the toes and differ from calluses in that corns have a sharply demarcated central core; corns can also develop between the toes and, due to the associated moisture, are often soft and macerated.

Calluses and corns are caused by a range of factors. These include ill-fitting footwear, bony prominences, malunited fractures, short or long metatarsals, and faulty foot biomechanics. The most common cause of calluses and corns in older people, particularly older women, is the wearing of shoes with a tight toebox (Frey et al. 1993; Frey 2000). It is likely that changing shoe-wearing habits would reduce the prevalence of hyperkeratotic lesions. However, it is difficult to change footwear behaviour—because fashion often outweighs practical considerations (Seale 1995).

Calluses and corns should be referred to a podiatrist—for debridement and enucleation of lesions using a scalpel. In most cases, this leads to immediate relief of pain, increases the bearable pressure threshold of the foot, and decreases the pressures borne by the metatarsal heads when walking. However, these benefits are generally only short-term, particularly if the underlying causes are not fully addressed. Longer-term management includes foot orthoses and surgery. However, the results of surgery are not always good, and surgery can be associated with 'transfer lesions'—the development of new lesions at previously lesion-free sites due to a post-operative alteration in foot mechanics.

There are several conservative techniques that can be used to decrease the rate at which the lesions re-form. Regular and frequent soaking of the feet, followed by mild rubbing with a pumice stone, can be very effective in keeping the lesions down to a bearable level.

There are also many over-the-counter products available. However, these should be selected with care. Simple foam-and-silicon pads offer effective temporary relief. However, medicated 'corn pads' should be avoided—because they contain acid preparations to break down the excessive build-up of skin.

Although this does not pose a problem for people with good skin integrity, it can cause problems, including ulceration, in people with frail skin and/or impaired peripheral vascular supply (such as older people with diabetes). When in doubt, nursing staff should consult a podiatrist.

Categories of foot problems

The following categories of foot problems are discussed in this chapter.

Nail disorders
- onychauxis (abnormal thickening of the nail)
- onychocryptosis ('ingrown' toenails)
- onychomycosis (fungal nail infections)
- other nail conditions (paronychia, onycholysis; onychomalacia, leukonychia, hippocratic nails)

Skin disorders
- hyperkeratosis (epidermal thickening—calluses and corns)

Structural foot problems
- hallux valgus (bunions)
- hallux limitus/rigidus (limited great toe movement)
- lesser-toe deformities (clawing, hammering, and retraction)

Functional foot problems
- abnormal mechanics of the foot when walking causing pain in the forefoot, arch, and heel

Structural foot problems

Nursing staff should be familiar with some of the more common foot deformities to ensure that they arrange timely and appropriate referral to footcare specialists. These deformities include: (i) hallux valgus; (ii) hallux limitus/rigidus; and (iii) lesser-toe deformities.

Hallux valgus

Hallux valgus, more commonly referred to as 'bunions', is the most common deformity of the foot. The term refers to an abnormal medial prominence of the first metatarsal head.

Although the most visible deformity is the bulbous (often inflamed) great toe joint, the condition often involves a progressive structural deformity of the entire forefoot. Hallux valgus is caused by many factors, including muscle imbalance, structural deformity of the metatarsals (which is sometimes an inherited trait), faulty foot mechanics, and the detrimental effects of ill-fitting footwear.

The enlarged first metatarsal head creates problems in finding suitable footwear, and the friction created by the shoe often leads to the formation of a bursa (fluid-filled sac) over the site. This can be extremely painful and, in older people with frail skin, can lead to ulceration.

Treatment of hallux valgus includes changing footwear to that with a broader forefoot, the application of foam or silicon pads over the joint, foot orthoses, and surgery. Surgery appears to provide better long-term results than orthoses (Torkki et al. 2001). However, there is a range of surgical techniques—and results vary. If surgery is considered, it is best to select a surgeon who specialises in foot surgery, because a specialist is more likely to choose the most appropriate technique for the presenting condition.

Hallux limitus/rigidus

Hallux limitus is a condition in which there is limited range of motion at the first metatarsophalangeal joint of the great toe. If this progresses to complete fusion of the joint, it is termed *hallux rigidus*. This condition is often very painful and can interfere with normal walking.

Treatment for hallux limitus involves foot orthoses to facilitate propulsion or manipulation, and injection with a corticosteroid. For hallux rigidus, surgery might be necessary. However, a large proportion of patients who change their footwear to that with a more ample toebox report good results, and this suggests that appropriate footwear is a sufficient treatment in many people (Smith, Katchis & Ayson 2000).

Lesser-toe deformity

Long-term wearing of ill-fitting footwear, in association with faulty foot mechanics and muscle weakness, can lead to the development of *lesser-toe deformities*. These include clawing, hammering, and retraction of the lesser toes.

Hammer toes and claw toes are among the most common foot complaints in older people, and can lead to the development of corns on the dorsum of the interphalangeal joints and calluses under the metatarsal heads.

Treatment involves footwear modification, various splinting devices, and management of the secondary lesions. Recurrent cases often require surgery to realign and stabilise the affected metatarsophalangeal or interphalangeal joints.

Functional foot problems

The term 'functional foot problems' refers to problems caused by abnormal mechanics of the foot when walking. These conditions can cause pain in the forefoot, arch, and heel.

Differentiating among these conditions requires careful diagnosis by footcare specialists. The role of nursing staff is to document the presence of any pain in the foot of the person, and to seek the opinion of a podiatrist. It is important to remember that foot pain should never be accepted as an inevitable aspect of ageing. Even chronic foot pain can be successfully managed by various conservative treatments.

> 'Foot pain should never be accepted as an inevitable aspect of ageing.'

Nursing considerations

Nurses are well placed to have a significant beneficial effect on the foot health of older people. Many foot problems can be diagnosed by nursing staff, and many potentially serious foot problems can be prevented by vigilant nursing care.

One of the most important, but least glamorous, aspects of older people nursing is the maintenance of good foot hygiene. Drying between the toes after showering can prevent excessive moisture build-up and decrease the risk of skin infection, and cutting the nails straight across (rather than into the corners) can prevent onychocryptosis (ingrown toenails).

Particular care needs to be taken with older people at risk of developing foot ulceration—such as people with diabetes mellitus, rheumatoid arthritis, or peripheral vascular disease. All breaches of the skin should be appropriately dressed, and the dressings should be changed frequently. Any sign of infection, such as swelling, erythema, or purulent discharge should be carefully noted and treated appropriately. The presence of hyperkeratotic lesions should not be ignored—because the lesion is often obscuring underlying skin break down.

Nursing role in foot care

Nurses are well placed to have a significant beneficial effect on the foot health of older people in their care. In particular, nurses can play a significant role in:
- vigilance, diagnosis, and referral of foot problems;
- foot hygeine;
- prevention of skin breakdown and ulceration; and
- education about appropriate footwear.

Nursing staff can significantly improve the foot health of those in their care by educating them about appropriate footwear. Inappropriate footwear contributes to a large proportion of foot problems in older people, and can be a significant factor in causing falls. Footwear design features to be noted include heel height, sole hardness, heel-collar height, and slip resistance of the sole. Older people should avoid very soft shoes, shoes with high heels, and shoes with slippery soles, but this can be difficult to implement. Many older people wear soft slippers because they are comfortable and easy to wash. However, 33% of older people who are admitted to hospital for a hip fracture were wearing slippers when they fell (Hourihan et al. 1997). Although it has not been proven that slippers are responsible for such falls, many slippers do incorporate two potentially hazardous features—in that they are soft and often have poor sole slip resistance.

'Nurses can significantly improve the foot health of those in their care by educating them about appropriate footwear.'

Nursing staff should therefore pay close attention to the shoes of older people. If they think that the shoes might be hazardous, nurses should educate the person (or a carer) regarding the features to look for when purchasing a new pair.

Conclusion

Although they are often overlooked, foot problems are one of the most important causes of impaired mobility in older people. Foot problems can be extremely painful and, in susceptible older people, they can lead to more serious conditions—such as ulceration, infection, and amputation.

Older people's nurses are well placed to prevent the development of some of these problems, to detect conditions that require treatment, and to refer older people to footcare specialists if necessary. Good foot health facilitates optimal mobility, and thus makes a significant contribution to the quality of life of older people.

'Good foot health facilitates mobility, and makes a significant contribution to the quality of life of older people.'

Chapter 6

Nutrition

Linda Kilworth

Introduction

Eating and drinking is basic to sustaining life. Withdrawing food and fluid leads to starvation and dehydration, and death ensues fairly quickly as bodily processes shut down due to lack of fuel and fluids. Due to the essential role of nutrition and hydration in sustaining life, nutrition should be a high priority in residential aged-care facilities. Most facilities have other clinical concerns that compete for priority, but clinical outcomes improve significantly when proper attention is paid to nutritional needs.

The simple provision of sufficient nutrients and energy will improve a person's health and general quality of life. The common problem of pressure ulcers illustrates the point. Dietary histories from people with pressure sores often reveal prolonged periods of poor food intake, especially meat. A person with a pressure ulcer will benefit from an

> 'Clinical outcomes improve significantly when proper attention is paid to nutritional needs.'

increase in high-value protein and vitamin C in his or her diet. Initial supplementation with a liquid protein formula will often result in improvements in wound healing over a few weeks. In addition, as dietary intake improves, the person becomes more alert and responsive and will often start eating better. Thus, both wound healing and quality of life are improved.

The principle that a good diet not only improves particular medical problems but also enhances general quality of life can be seen in most residents of care homes. People are often admitted to such facilities because they are frail and unable to look after themselves. Many have not been able to consume a nutritionally sound diet—often through lack of motivation and a diminished interest in living. After an initial settling-in period (during which the person has to face the realities of a reduction in independence and an increased awareness of the frailty of ageing), new residents can gain weight, control their blood glucose levels better, and generally show marked improvement in overall health. Careful management of the foods and fluids that are offered can alleviate a range of problems— including constipation, infections, weight loss, confusion, vitamin deficiency (such as scurvy), diverticular disease, and other nutrition-related illnesses.

'A good diet not only improves particular medical problems but also enhances general quality of life.'

Nutritional assessment

When a person is admitted to a care home, it is important to: (i) assess whether a nutritional problem exists; and (ii) develop management strategies to combat any problems that do exist.

Nutrition-related problems can be identified by using a screening-and-assessment tool. However, most of these are in the form of questionnaires, and many residents are often unable to complete such tools accurately. It is usually easier (and more accurate) to observe food and fluid intake over a period of time. This can be monitored using a food-and-fluid chart. The charts need to be user-friendly, because staff members often have little time to complete a detailed form. A useful form consists simply of a list of foods that reflect the items on the menu, together with a column to record the amount of food that is eaten by the person. An example is given in Table 6.1 (page 65).

Table 6.1 A simple food-and-fluid assessment chart

Food and fluid	Quantity eaten/offered	Other comments
Breakfast		
Cereal (wheat biscuit)	1 biscuit	biscuit eaten, but prefers porridge
Milk	half-jug	
Toast	two slices offered	refused
Tea	1 cup	with 2 sugars and milk

Author's creation

The 'Comments' column is useful to obtain a profile of residents' likes and dislikes. Determining this is important because most residents are reluctant to ask for different foods or for more foods (Pearson, FitzGerald & Nay 2003). In addition, carers will often impose their own preferences on the people whom they assist with feeding (Pearson, FitzGerald & Nay 2003). If a carer likes a particular food or dish, that food is likely to be served first. If the carer likes to put a little bit of several foods onto his or her fork, the carer will engage in a similar practice when feeding other people. In contrast, the person being fed might prefer to eat each food item separately, or might like to eat all food covered in tomato sauce or Worcestershire sauce. These individual eating styles can be recorded in the 'Comments' column of an assessment chart, and thus be relayed to other carers. The simple procedure of offering food in a style that is desirable to the person will encourage eating.

The 'Comments' column can also record other observations—such as the fact that a relative brought food for a person, that this was consumed shortly before a meal, and, consequently, that the person consumed less food at a particular meal.

Two basic questions

In the final analysis, nutritional assessment can be simplified to two basic questions.
• Is the resident eating and drinking enough food?
• Is the resident losing weight?

If the answer the first question is 'no', and the answer to the second question is 'yes', the problem should be investigated further.

If a pattern develops that indicates a person is consuming high-energy, low-nutrient foods at the expense of the nutritious meals provided by the care home, the person can be counselled. In addition, the issue can be discussed at case conferences with relatives and friends, and strategies can be developed.

Anthropometric measures

The usual methods used to determine current nutritional status are: (i) measuring height and weight; (ii) evaluating biochemical data; and (iii) observing weight loss or gains over a period of time.

Measuring height is necessary to assess whether weight is appropriate. Height is difficult to measure in some people, especially those with kyphosis or other spinal deformities. Those who can stand can be measured against the wall. Difficulties can also be experienced in assessing height in bed-bound persons. There are several methods that can be used. These include:

▶ *recumbent bed height*—the person is measured in bed with a tape measure;
▶ *demi span*—a measure is taken from the middle of the sternal notch to the second webspace of the hand; the person's height can then be calculated using separate formulae for males and females; and
▶ *knee height*—the person's knees are bent and a measure is taken from the heel to the kneecap; a formula is again used to calculate height.

Most residents (and some relatives) can give an estimate of their height when they were younger. This is often a good estimate, and involves less stress for the resident.

Weight

Weight losses or gains are a good indicator of nutritional status. Food intake often declines with age, and unintentional weight losses are common. Decreased food intake can be due to age-related anorexia, appetite loss through depression or drugs, dysphagia, or metabolic changes through infections. Diseases such as Parkinson's disease, Huntington's chorea, and dementia (especially in association with wandering or excessive involuntary movements) produce a higher metabolic expenditure and require more energy to prevent weight loss.

Monitoring weight is essential for early detection of weight loss. Weight stabilisation (or gain) can then be achieved by changing feeding techniques and offering a high-energy, high-protein diet.

'Monitoring weight is essential for early detection of weight loss.'

Residents should therefore be weighed monthly—preferably at the same time of day, in approximately the same clothes, using the same set of scales. These weights should be recorded. The best method is to present the data in graphical format because it is easier to observe upwards or downwards trends in weight. This method allows staff members to note small weight losses regularly over an extended period of time. The Box below shows how regular careful checks can be useful in detecting a potentially significant weight loss that might have otherwise gone unnoticed.

Noting a trend

Regular weight checks, and recording of the findings, can be useful in detecting small (but potentially significant) weight loss.

A man who originally weighed 86 kg was losing, on average, 0.75 kg per month. This weight loss (of less than 1 kg per month) might seem to be minor. However, if this were to continue, this man would lose 9 kg in a year. This represents 10% of his usual body weight. Such a weight loss would be significant. By measuring his weight monthly, and recording the results graphically, nursing staff were able to detect the trend and take appropriate steps.

An unintentional weight loss of this magnitude over a period of time should be noted and acted upon. More significantly, a weight loss of 1–2 kg in any one month is of immediate concern, and strategies should be instigated to prevent further weight losses.

The best measure for assessing appropriate weight is the body mass index (BMI) (NHMRC 1999). BMI is calculated as follows:

BMI = weight (kg)/height (m)^2

For example, using the above formula, a person of 2 m height who weighed 50 kg would have a BMI of:

$50/2^2 = 50/4 = 12.5$

This person would therefore have a BMI of 12.5. Recommended BMIs are as shown in Table 6.2 (page 68).

In the example given above, the person with a calculated BMI of 12.5 would therefore be considered underweight.

It is difficult to assess the weight of bedridden residents who cannot be weighed on a set of scales. Taking the mid-arm circumference of the upper arm is a useful way of approximating weight. Using various formulae, total body weight can then be calculated using the mid-arm circumference measure and knee height.

Table 6.2 Recommended BMIs

BMI	Recommendation
<20	Underweight
20–25	Acceptable weight
25–30	Overweight
>30	Obese

Author's creation

Eating patterns and behaviours
Institutional changes to eating patterns

Everyone has different eating patterns. Before entering a care home, many older people might have been familiar with eating their main hot meal in the evening. However, they might now be faced with eating the hot meal at midday. This is just one example of how institutions require residents to change their eating patterns to fit in with the facility's functional need to provide meals efficiently. Some residents find these changes difficult, and their food intake can be reduced as a result.

Variation in diet can also be a problem. In their own homes, people have the option of varying their diets by eating out or by purchasing take-aways. This is usually not possible in the residential environment, but the monotony of a set cyclical menu can be alleviated by offering outings to family restaurants, picnics, and theme days. Increasing residents' enjoyment of food will increase food intake.

> 'Increasing residents' enjoyment of food will increase food intake.'

Individual abilities and behaviours

At the time of admission to the care home or if a resident's clinical condition deteriorates, it is important to assess the person's ability to feed with a knife and fork, drink from a cup, and chew and swallow foods. If a person's ability to self-feed deteriorates, less food will be consumed, and malnourishment can become a problem. Assistance with feeding will be required.

For some people, ageing results in a functional decline, but not necessarily a cognitive deterioration. In these circumstances, some people find it difficult to acknowledge that they have lost the ability to feed themselves. Sometimes, through pride or sheer stubbornness, people can refuse assistance. Staff members need to show empathy in these circumstances, and assist residents to accept these changes.

Other behaviours that can cause difficulties include:

▶ hoarding or pilfering food (which can lead to weight gains, sometimes excessive);
▶ refusing the meal presented, or walking away from the table;
▶ spending a long time eating food; and
▶ antisocial behaviour at mealtimes.

Environmental issues such as too much noise, too little light, too much glare, cluttered tables, and inappropriate seating arrangements can exacerbate behavioural problems.

It is important to discuss needs with residents in an attempt to resolve these issues. Sometimes the solution is surprisingly simple—such as placing the person in one corner of the dining-room, with a window view, and with no other person at the table. Although this might seem to be isolating the person, such a solution is often workable and satisfactory for all concerned.

Nutritional issues in aged-care facilities
Malnutrition

Malnutrition, which is characterised by weight loss and muscle-wasting, is caused by inadequate intake of energy and nutrients. Factors such as not eating or drinking enough food and fluids, vomiting, diarrhoea, fever, and excessive involuntary movements can cause energy and nutrient losses and, over a prolonged period, will lead to malnutrition.

It is sometimes difficult to decide whether refusing food and fluid is a natural part of the dying process, or a response to ill-health and pain. However, alleviating pain and ensuring that the person is comfortable will often encourage eating.

'Alleviating pain and ensuring that the person is comfortable will often encourage eating.'

Many people will cease eating long before they stop drinking. Providing high-energy, high-protein beverages can reverse the anorexia, and the person will often start to eat again. Staff should continue to offer food and fluids, even if these are repeatedly refused. Occasionally, the person will accept a meal, or eat some food. Small amounts of food offered frequently, and presented attractively, are more acceptable than three large meals a day. However, the daily schedules in many facilities are not flexible enough to allow people to eat in this fashion.

It is important to 'make every mouthful count'. This can be achieved by offering only foods and fluids that have some nutritional value. The Box below provides some suggestions.

'Making every mouthful count'

To help to minimise malnutrition, nurses should 'make every mouthful count' by offering foods of high nutritional value. Suggestions include:

- milk shakes;
- dairy desserts;
- fortified custards;
- fortified cereals (some people can manage milky cereals several times a day);
- yoghurt; and
- fortified soups (soaked with bread pieces).

Commercially available supplements are often useful. These are available in various forms and flavours.

Dehydration

Dehydration is essentially a decrease in fluid intake and/or an increase in fluid loss. Older people have reduced thirst sensation, decreased renal function, and a smaller proportion of body water. Many older people also have an aversion to drinking large volumes of fluid—perhaps due to concerns about urinary incontinence, or the possibility of unwanted nocturnal urination.

Rapid weight loss can be an indication of dehydration, but this is not a definitive guide. Nurses should check for physical signs and symptoms of dehydration such as dryness of the lips, conjunctiva, and mucous membranes, decreased salivary and bronchial secretions, sunken eyeballs, fever, postural hypotension, nausea, constipation, decreased appetite, weight loss, loss of elasticity of the skin, and disorientation. Dehydration can also cause or increase confusion.

Dehydration is a risk-management issue, and every facility should continuously assess its risk. It is important that staff members be in the habit of 'pushing fluids', and that regular fluid rounds be part of the routine.

Steps that can be taken to minimise the risk of deydration are listed in the Box on page 71.

Minimising the risk of dehydration

Steps that can be taken to prevent dehydration include the following.

- Aim for 30 millilitres of fluid per kilogram of body weight per day, with a minimum of 1500 millilitres per day. This can be any fluid, not only water.
- Plan the menu to include items with higher fluid content (for example, soups, casseroles, jelly-based desserts, ice cream, and ice blocks).
- Encourage staff members to offer sips of beverage each time they are close to residents, or whenever they enter the room.
- Encourage variety in fluids (for example, tea, coffee, milk, fruit juices, soups, water). If weight loss is a problem, ensure that the beverages offered are high in energy and nutrients.
- Some 'sports' or 'electrolyte' drinks are absorbed easily and can be useful for some people
- The temperature of fluids that are offered should be carefully considered because some people like very cold water (perhaps with ice), whereas others prefer water at room temperature.
- Offer extra thickened fluids because some thickening agents reduce the amount of available free water. Staff should be encouraged to offer thickened fluids in the evenings and early mornings.

Dysphagia

Dysphagia (difficulty with swallowing) is associated with a variety of conditions—including strokes, dementia, multiple sclerosis, motor neurone disease, Parkinson's disease, and cancer of the mouth and throat. Because of the physical difficulties associated with swallowing, it is safer to offer people with dysphagia a texture-modified diet. The swallowing assessment should be conducted by a speech pathologist who will assess the difficulty in terms of the three stages of swallowing. Once this has been determined, food and fluid consistency can be modified.

Texture-modified foods are not indicated for people who are slow eaters. Rather, they are designed to overcome the real physical difficulties and dangers associated with dysphagia. Such foods can prevent choking or aspiration, and they should therefore not be perceived disparagingly by staff members. If carers make comments such as 'mush',

'Texture-modified foods can prevent choking or aspiration, and they should not be perceived disparagingly by staff members.'

'baby food', or 'goo', this sends a message to the resident that the food is unappealing. Many will refuse to eat it (and no wonder!).

Things to consider are:

▶ the temperature of the meal; if a meal is cold, it can be unpalatable;

▶ the taste; mincing food will decrease flavour, particularly if the meal is held for a period of time;

▶ taste preferences; people will refuse meals that do not appeal to their taste;

▶ small frequent meals; such meals accommodate slow eaters;

▶ positioning; try to position the person in a way that makes eating and swallowing comfortable;

▶ independence; encourage independence by using appropriate plates, utensils, and drinking equipment.

Texture-modified diets

Types of texture-modified diets

There are four general categories of texture-modified foods. These are listed in the Box below.

Types of texture-modified diets

The four types of texture-modified diets are as follows.

Normal texture or full diet

No modification

Soft texture or cut-up moist foods

Stews; casseroles; soft vegetables and fruit; extra gravy or sauce

Minced texture

Ground meat; minced or mashed vegetables; stewed fruits; extra gravy or sauce

Puréed or smooth texture

Liquefied; no lumps; smooth consistency, but not runny; extra gravy or sauce

---

Often residents can manage texture combinations—such as minced meats and well-cooked vegetables; or puréed meat with mashed vegetables. Sauces and gravies are essential to keep food moist.

Residents on texture-modified diets are at greater risk of malnutrition

> 'Residents on texture-modified diets are at greater risk of malnutrition.'

because the addition of liquid, when blending the food down into a smooth paste, reduces the nutrients per volume. This risk is especially high with puréed or smooth-texture foods. Using milk, gravy, white sauce, and other high-energy liquids helps. Supplements are often required as a precaution and as extra energy.

Breads and cereals are low in texture-modified diets. Nurses should therefore consider:

▶ adding bread pieces or bread crumbs when puréeing food;
▶ blending cereal with milk and sugar to form a paste; and
▶ blending milk or custard with crustless bread that has been soaked in milk. Offering these between meals will help to keep the energy value high.

Presentation of texture-modified diets

The 'sameness' of presentation of these modified textures is enough to reduce the appetite of many residents. Nurses should try to make texture-modified foods attractive and appealing. Some suggestions are as follows.

▶ Use different crockery. For example, meat and potatoes can be presented in a small ramekin with vegetables on the side. Desserts can be served in a parfait glass. Mousse with cream looks better in a parfait glass than in a dessert bowl.
▶ Pipe the food onto the plate using a piping bag, rather than using a scoop.
▶ Moulds can make interesting shapes on the plate.
▶ Make a vegetable terrine and slice it so that it looks different.
▶ Some foods can be placed in a round pie dish and sliced in wedges.

Thickened fluids

Many of these diets are accompanied by thickened fluids. Several levels of thickened fluids can be made up, depending on the severity of the swallowing problem.

It is important to vary the flavour of these fluids throughout the day. Offering lime cordial for the whole day is unappealing (especially if lime is not a favourite flavour!). Apart from taste, it is important to assess these thickened fluids for the level of hydration that they offer.

Many thickening agents are now commercially available. There are two basic types:

▶ modified starches—these can be used in both hot and cold beverages; and
▶ gums—guar gum, xanthan gum, and carrageen gum are most often used. Thickening agents can also be used in beer and wine.

Some fluids that do not require thickening can be offered. These include fruit nectars, dairy desserts, custards, yoghurts, thick soups, and instant puddings. These are often better tolerated because some thickening agents leave an after-taste that residents dislike.

Finger foods

Finger foods (that is, foods that can be picked up and eaten with the fingers) are good for people with dementia who have a diminished ability to use utensils. Finger foods are a way of promoting independent eating and will result in an increase in energy and nutrient consumption.

It is important that finger foods are nutritious. High-fat, high-salt commercial varieties (such as mini-pies and sausage rolls) should be avoided. Foods in wrappers and foil, and foods containing pips, seeds, or bones are not suitable.

Some suggestions for nutritious finger foods are listed in the Box below.

Nutritious finger foods

Some suggestions for nutritious finger foods are
- toasted fingers;
- sandwiches (cut into fingers, pinwheels, or ribbons);
- asparagus and ham rolls;
- savoury scones;
- fish, chicken, or meatballs;
- cut-up fruit;
- blanched vegetables (cut up into finger portions);
- wedges of cheese;
- vegetable fritters or tempura;
- small slices of quiche; and
- antipasto plate.

Therapeutic diets

Therapeutic diets can be very restrictive and can reduce the appetite of some people. They can also compromise optimal nutrition. Therapeutic diets are therefore beneficial in care homes only if there is a clear clinical advantage to the resident—for example, lactose-free diets for those who have lactose intolerance.

Other therapeutic diets that are beneficial include:
- diabetic diets—these generally follow healthy eating guidelines, and can incorporate some sugar;
- gluten-free diets—to reduce symptoms of coeliac disease;
- vegetarian diets—usually due to long-term personal preference;
- specific food allergies—eliminating known allergens; and
- renal diets—to assist in maintaining kidney function.

Menu-planning

The menu must be enjoyable, provide reasonable choice, provide sufficient variety, and meet the nutritional needs of the residents. If these factors are not accounted for when designing a menu, residents will not eat the food, wastage will be high, and residents will look for other sources of food (or go hungry).

Table 6.3 Example of a daily menu template

Meal	Suggestions
Breakfast	cereal, porridge, or semolina milk and/or yoghurt choice of breads; toast with butter or margarine and spreads fruit and/or fruit juice cooked meal beverage
Midday meal	main dishmeat, poultry, seafood, egg gravy or sauce (these assist swallowing) 1 starchy vegetable such as potato, or substitute rice, pasta, cous cous, polenta 2 or 3 green or yellow vegetables dessert: milk-based, fruit-based, or both beverage
Evening meal	soup (add vegetables, barley, rice, bread, lentils) choice of bread or bread rolls with butter/margarine hot main dish (can be finger-food option) 1 or 2 vegetables OR sandwich (specific to resident's request) or toasted sandwich OR protein item (ham, egg, cheese, chicken, tuna) with salad fruit or dessert beverage

Mid morning, mid afternoon, and late evening	healthy options include quarter-sandwiches, ribbon sandwiches,
	   fruit buns, toast, yoghurt, dairy dessert, cheese and biscuits,
	   biscuit and dip, sliced fruit, pikelets, fruit balls, custard, even
	   breakfast cereal with milk
	offer cake, slice, muffins, scones, and biscuits once a day
	   beverage

Author's creation

Good menu-planning also involves consideration of the kitchen facilities and equipment, the type of operation (cook-fresh or cook-chill), the skills of the kitchen staff, and the budget. The menu should also consider any cultural or religious requirements.

An example of a daily menu template that is nutritionally balanced is shown in Table 6.3 (page 75).

It is important to note that breakfast is often the best-eaten meal of the day. Items offered at breakfast are familiar to most residents, particularly those on texture-modified diets, and there is usually a variety of choices. The nutrition of residents can be increased by offering a hot breakfast with a high protein content.

> 'Breakfast is often the best-eaten meal of the day.'

It is essential to offer and encourage a late-evening snack, particularly for diabetics. This allows for better blood glucose control and prevents early wakening and restlessness due to hunger.

It is good practice in planning menus to include foods that can be easily modified for various textures—so that the overall workload is lessened. Nurses should try to avoid using the texture-modified midday meal leftovers in the evening. People do not usually appreciate two meals that are exactly the same each day.

A cyclical menu should be at least three weeks long. However, most establishments find four weeks easier to manage. As a general rule, there should be no repetition of dishes throughout the menu—unless the majority of residents request it or it is required for religious or traditional requirements. Fish, for example is often served on Fridays and on Ash Wednesday. If fish is served on Fridays, nurses should try to vary the dishes each week throughout the cycle. For example, crumbed fish can be served in the first week, fish cakes in the second week, fish in a beer batter in the third week, and smoked cod with white sauce in the fourth week.

When preparing the menu, it is best to list the roast dishes (for example, roast chicken, beef, lamb, pork, veal, continental pot roast) that will be offered. These should be placed on different days of each week—to prevent one day of the week being recognised as a 'roast day'. A list should then be made of all other dishes that are to be included on the menu. These can be inserted into each week using the menu template. Dishes should be placed into the menu template such that similar dishes are not repeated on consecutive days. Similar meats or flavours should not be offered on consecutive days.

The placement of dishes on the Sunday of week four and the Monday of week one should be carefully considered. In a cyclical menu, these days follow each other.

Once all main dishes are placed in the menu cycle, the accompaniments (such as the potato or starch dishes, vegetables, and desserts) can be added. Nurses should try to avoid repetition of flavours. For example, corned beef with a white sauce and potato bake are similar in flavour. Nurses should try to imagine what the food will look like when presented on the plate. For example, chicken in a white sauce with mashed potato and cauliflower would present as an all-white meal and look very unappealing. Imagine the colour when minced or puréed!

Once the basic template of main meals is completed, the evening meal items can be inserted. Ensure there is no repetition of flavours in one day and on consecutive days. For example, if beef was served at the midday meal, serve pork or fish for the evening meal.

Principles of menu-planning

The main principles of menu-planning include the following:
* consideration of the kitchen facilities and equipment;
* awareness of cultural or religious requirements;
* awareness that breakfast is often the best-eaten meal of the day;
* offering and encouraging a late-evening snack;
* including foods that can be easily modified for various textures;
* establishing a cyclical menu;
* taking advantage of seasonal items;
* assessing the popularity of the menu; and
* enhancing flavour to avoid blandness in foods offered.

Try to take advantage of seasonal items. These are usually cheaper and at peak quality. Changing menus to reflect seasons is also encouraged. Offering more cool desserts in summer is more appealing than hot steamed puddings. Many facilities start from 'scratch' to design seasonal menus. However, in reality, these can be recycled each season, with the addition of two or three new menu items.

It is important to assess the popularity of the menu—either through formal surveys or simply by noting dining-room wastage. Wastage is a good indicator of menu-item popularity, and it can also provide

> 'It is important to assess the popularity of the menu . . . Wastage is a good indicator of menu-item popularity,'

information on the adequacy of meal sizes. Meal sizes should be flexible to accommodate the smallest eater and those who like large full plates.

Residents often complain the food is bland and tasteless. Adding extra salt is not the solution. Nurses should try to enhance flavours by:

- adding concentrated stock to wet dishes, soups, and vegetables;
- adding citrus juices, pineapple juice, pickles, vinegar, sweet-and-sour sauces, lemonade and bitters; tart flavours are well accepted;
- adding bacon pieces, ham strips, onion;
- adding wine, beer, or mayonnaise to soups and sauces;
- marinating meat, chicken, and fish in alcohol, soy sauce, commercial marinades, fruit juices, or a demi-glace sauce;
- using strong herbs (but care should be taken if using a cook-chill system because herbs have a tendency to become over-powering when food is left to stand for some time); and
- using appropriate temperatures; that is, serving hot foods hot and cold foods cold to enhance flavour.

Conclusion

Careful management of nutritional and hydration needs provides residents with better quality of life and enhances staff morale.

Good management begins with accurate assessment of individual residents and consideration of their particular nutritional issues.

Good menu-planning, an efficient food-service department, and regular monitoring and review will all assist in ensuring that residents of Care Homes are well nourished and hydrated.

Chapter 7
Enteral Feeding

Patsy Montgomery

Introduction

In caring for older people who are unable to eat or swallow oral foods, nurses and carers must ensure that the appropriate nutritional requirements are met. These nutritional goals are set by a multidisciplinary team, including (depending on circumstances) the person's doctor, dietitian, speech therapist, nurses, carers, and family.

Definitions and indications

Enteral feeding is the supply of liquid nutrients via a tube into the gastro-intestinal tract, bypassing the mouth and oesophagus.

The liquid nutrients go directly into:

▶ the stomach through a gastrostomy tube—also called a 'G tube' or 'percutaneous endoscopic gastrostomy' (PEG);

▶ the jejunum (a section of the small intestine) through a jejunostomy tube—also called a 'J tube'; or

▶ the stomach or jejunum via a nasogastric tube or a nasojejunal tube (not commonly used for the elderly).

The indications and contraindications for enteral feeding are listed in the Box below.

Indications and contraindications for enteral feeding

Indications

The indications for enteral feeding include:
- dysphagia (difficulty with swallowing) due to dysfunction of the swallowing reflex;
- dysphagia due to neurological impairment (for example, stroke or cerebral palsy);
- dysphagia or obstruction due to tumour;
- unconscious state; and
- HIV/AIDS.

Contraindications

The contraindications for enteral feeding include:
- non-functioning gut;
- morbid obesity;
- cardiovascular instability;
- oesophageal reflux
- ascites.

Nutritional assessment

In assessing a person's nutritional status, the first decision to be made is whether it is stable, deteriorating, or improving. In making this assessment, and in identifying the person's specific nutritional problems, nurses should take into account the nature of the person's illness, the past medical history, and the relevant social and nutritional history.

Other factors to be considered include anthropometric data—such as height, weight, skinfold thickness, and arm circumference. Weight loss of 10% or more over a 3-month period is a good indication of an inadequate energy intake. Biomedical data should also be taken into account. This might include haemoglobin, total lymphocyte count, electrolyte levels, and albumin.

'Weight loss of 10% or more over a 3-month period is a good indication of an inadequate energy intake.'

Placement of the tube

The tube can be placed in position using an endoscope. If the tube is placed in the stomach (through the skin), the technique is called percutaneous endoscopic gastrostomy (PEG). If placed in the jejunum, it is called percutaneous endoscopic jejunostomy (PEJ). Alternatively, radiography or fluoroscopy using X-rays can be used to guide the tube into the correct position.

The placement of the initial tube requires a short visit to an endoscopy unit or day surgery unit, following which the person often returns to residential accommodation on the same day. Nursing staff should therefore be aware of the nursing requirements for these people upon their return. Particular attention should be paid to the following:

▶ peristomal skin care;
▶ documentation; and
▶ observations.

With respect to *peristomal skin care*, nurses can expect a haemoserous discharge around the insertion site for 24–48 hours. This should be cleaned with normal saline, dried, and covered with gauze. Initially, this should be performed twice daily, and then as required. It can be ceased when the area is dry.

Documentation should include a record of the type and size of the tube and skin-level marking. Tube tension should be noted, and if a balloon tube is in use the amount of water in the balloon should be noted.

Nurses should *observe* the wound area for inflammation, tenderness, drainage, and possible tube migration.

For more information on the longer-term care of the site and tube, see 'Caring for the tube site', this chapter, page 83.

Feeding

Enteral feeding is initiated after discussion with the dietitian, and can commence 6–12 hours after insertion of the tube. The matters to be decided include: (i) the type of delivery; and (ii) the type of formula.

Type of delivery

The choice of the form of delivery of enteral feeding depends on the tolerance and absorption rate of the recipient. There are three main forms of delivery:

▶ *syringe or bolus feeding*: in this form of delivery, the formula is administered using a 60-millilitre catheter-tipped syringe;
▶ *gravity feeding*: in this case, the formula is delivered using a container and a giving set suspended from an intravenous (IV) pole above the person;

the formula flows by gravity and is regulated with a roller clamp; and

▶ *pump feeding:* in this case, the formula is delivered accurately by a mechanical pump, which allows rate and dose to be set.

With all forms of delivery, the tube should be flushed with 30–50 millilitres of tap water after feeding.

Type of formula

The choice of the type of formula is within the domain of the dietitian. In making this decision, the dietitian will make the following assessments of the person: (i) nutritional needs (such as fluid, energy, and protein requirements); (ii) clinical condition; (iii) metabolic profile; and (iv) tolerance to the feed.

The feeding management should be reviewed as required, especially if the person loses weight, or experiences vomiting, diarrhoea, or reflux.

Commercially produced enteral formulae are convenient and sterile, and have a known composition. There is a wide variety available to accommodate different needs. They come in two types:

▶ powders, which mix with water and are cheaper, but which require time and labour to reconstitute; and

▶ liquids, which come in 'ready-to-use' cans or 'ready-to-hang' pre-filled containers.

These formulae contain protein, fat, and carbohydrate in the required proportions. Vitamins, minerals, and electrolytes are added, as required, to give a complete feed. The recommended dietary intake (RDI) on the container indicates the nutrient benefits to be obtained from a given volume of each feed. The categories of formulae are shown in the Box below.

Categories of formulae

Formulae can be categorised as follows:

- *iso-osmolar:* the most commonly used feeds; well tolerated and readily available;
- *hyper-osmolar:* nutrients in a more concentrated solution; for people with high energy needs or those who have fluid restrictions;
- *fibre-added:* formulae with fibre added to assist with bowel function;
- *elemental:* formulae that require minimal or no digestion;
- *disease-specific:* custom-designed formulae to meet special needs (for example, products for people with renal disease contain low protein, low fluid, and modified mineral and electrolyte content);
- *single-nutrient source:* preparations of protein, fat, and carbohydrate available separately; can be added to existing formulae.

In assessing a person's dietary requirements and the type of enteral feed to be used, blood tests can be ordered to determine urea, electrolytes, albumin, total protein, creatinine, and blood glucose levels. After an initial assessment and stabilisation, biochemistry should be sought at least every six months to check for urea, electrolytes, albumin, and total protein. For diabetics, once the condition is stable, random blood glucose levels should be checked and recorded as needed.

Caring for the tube site

The tube site should be checked every day, and daily cleaning of the tube site is essential to prevent infection. A bath or shower is a good opportunity to wash around the area and under the external flange, using a washer or gauze. Warm water should be used, together with a skin-cleansing gel to clean the area.

> 'The tube site should be checked every day, and daily cleaning of the tube site is essential to prevent infection.'

Dressings are not required, but a small gauze dressing can be used to protect the clothing. A small amount of serous ooze around the tube site is normal, and this might make the skin somewhat red. This is not a cause for concern. However, the nurse should note if there is any significant redness, especially if this is observed in association with pain or tenderness, swelling, or any unusual drainage around the tube (such as bloody, malodorous, or formula-like fluid). If there is pus around the site, the nurse should take a swab for culture and organise appropriate antibiotics.

Granulation tissue (or 'proud flesh') is often present. Unless it is painful there is no point in removing such granulation tissue—because it is likely to grow back again.

The external disc can sometimes be too tight against the external abdominal wall—causing blanching. The disc can be released by gently pushing away from the abdominal wall. About 1–2 centimetres of 'in–out play' should be allowed. A net abdominal stocking or cotton cummerbund can be used to keep the tube in place.

Nurses should be aware that swimming is not detrimental to the site.

Administration of medications

Most medications can be given through the gastrostomy tube, but nurses should use liquid medications whenever possible or crush tablets into a fine powder and mix well in warm water. The nurse should check with the doctor or pharmacist regarding the availability of liquid forms of medication, and to ensure that it is appropriate to crush tablets. In particular, care should be taken with enteric-coated or time-release tablets, which should not usually be crushed.

The medication should not be mixed with the formula, and medications should not be mixed together. The tube should be flushed with 30 millilitres of warm water before and after giving each medication (flushing between each medication if there are multiple medications to be administered).

If a jejunostomy tube is in situ, nurses should check with the doctor or pharmacist that the medication will be absorbed in the small intestine—because the stomach and duodenum are bypassed by a jejunostomy tube.

Venting or decompression

Abdominal discomfort and bloating can be caused by excessive air or gas in the stomach. Allowing the air to escape is called 'venting' or 'decompression'. The venting process takes only a couple of minutes, and can be carried out before feeding, or as required.

If the person has a PEG or gastronomy tube with a balloon, the nurse should remove the cap from the feeding port and attach a 60-millilitre syringe (barrel only) to the feeding port. The syringe should be lowered to a position below the stomach. The contents and air (froth and bubbles) can then be allowed to fill the syringe. The fluid contents can be drained back into the stomach by raising the syringe above the stomach.

If the person has a low-profile device (stomate), these devices have a non-reflux valve in the tip of the tube, which stops the stomach contents refluxing up the tube and spilling from the feeding port. A decompression tube can be inserted into the stomate, which opens the non-reflux valve and allows the air to escape.

In the case of low-profile devices with a balloon, nurses should be aware that these devices have a non-reflux valve at the entry of the tube. The nurse should connect the straight extension tube to the feeding port, attach a 60-millilitre catheter-tipped syringe to the extension tube, and lower the syringe below the stomach. As with the PEG, the contents and air can be allowed to fill the syringe, and then the fluid contents can be drained back into the stomach by raising the syringe above the stomach.

General care

Cleaning the equipment

Containers, gravity feeding sets, pump sets, and syringes should all be washed in warm, soapy water, rinsed in warm water, and patted dry. They should then be stored in a clean, covered container or wrapped in a clean towel until the next use. In hotter climates, they should be stored in a refrigerator.

In acute hospitals the equipment is changed every 24 hours, or as recommended by the manufacturing company. In the community, in nursing homes, and at home, the equipment should be changed twice weekly.

Weight

Keeping a record of the person's weight will help to determine if weight goals are being met. This is very difficult if the person is non-ambulant. In these cases, observation of any body changes will help in making assessments.

Nurses should discuss the situation with the dietitian if they have any concerns about the person's body weight.

Mouth care

Effective mouth care is essential in preventing dental caries. Effective mouth care continues to be important in people who are not taking food orally. Those who are able to attend to their own care should be encouraged to brush their teeth and use a mouthwash. For those who are unable to brush their teeth, nurses can attend to mouth care using a foam-tipped applicator with toothpaste or mouthwash. A face cloth can be used to wipe the teeth and gums. A spray can be used to keep the mouth moist, and a moisturising cream can be used for the lips. A detailed discussion of mouth care is given in Chapter 3.

Feeding position

The head should be raised 30 degrees (in a 'semi-Fowler's' position) when the person is sitting in a chair or propped up in bed. The person should not be isolated while feeding, and some interaction is required. As with mealtimes for other people, feeding is a social time of the day for those who are reliant on enteral feeding.

> 'The person should not be isolated . . . feeding is a social time of the day for those who are reliant on enteral feeding.'

Checking tube position

The position of the tube should be checked before feeding by recording the measurement of the skin disc against the calibrations (numbers) on the tube. (If numbers are not present, an indelible pen can be used to mark the tube's correct position.) The figure as measured before each feeding should be compared with previous measurements. If there is a significant difference, this should be reported.

Troubleshooting

Blocked tube

If the feeding tube becomes blocked and the flow is slow or stops, the following method can be used to unblock it.

- Insert a 30–60-millilitre syringe in the end port of the tube.
- Pull back the plunger and withdraw as much fluid as possible from the tube. Discard any fluid aspirated.
- Reinsert the syringe with 10–20 millilitres of warm water and move the plunger back and forth.
- If the tube does not clear, leave the water in the tube and clamp the tube for 10 minutes and try again.
- Notify the senior staff member on duty if unable to clear the blockage.

Ben

Ben, a 76-year-old man with a stroke, who lived in a nursing home had had a PEG for six months. He had suffered from consistent diarrhoea for a few months. Examination of his history revealed that the delivery of the formula had been changed from a gravity feed (which took 40 minutes) to a bolus feed with a syringe. It is very difficult to do a bolus feed slowly, and the formula was going in too quickly for Ben to tolerate. Too much formula too quickly can cause diarrhoea.

When the nursing staff reverted to a gravity feed, Ben began to miss out on activities because he was always attached to a gravity set. The staff decided to try a feeding pump overnight, followed by a top up during the day. This freed Ben to do the activities he wanted during the day, and proved to be very successful—not only for Ben but also for the staff.

Diarrhoea

Diarrhoea could be due to:

- medications;
- bacterial contamination of the equipment;

▶ impaction of faeces; or

▶ incorrect delivery of the formula—that is too much formula too quickly.

The person's past medical history should be checked, and steps should be taken to ascertain the cause and manage appropriately. The story of Ben (Box, page 86) illustrates the successful management of this problem.

Constipation

There will be a change in bowel habits once a PEG is placed in situ, and it is not uncommon for the bowels to open only twice per week if using a standard formula. However, nursing staff should check with a dietitian regarding any significant change in bowel habits.

Constipation could be due to:

▶ medications;

▶ change in diet; or

▶ reduced fluid intake.

Again, the person's past medical history should be checked, and steps should be taken to ascertain the cause and manage appropriately. The story of Mary (Box, below) illustrates the successful management of this problem.

Mary

Mary was an 83-year-old woman who had suffered a stroke. After treatment in an acute hospital, she was discharged to a nursing home. A PEG was placed in situ because she suffered from dysphagia and had a limited gag reflex. Mary was non-ambulant and had very little use of her limbs.

The nurses were concerned that Mary's bowels opened only twice a week, and that her stools were of a hard consistency. The nurses checked with Mary's family and found that she had previously lived alone and that her diet had usually consisted of a cup of tea and toast. She ate very little fibre and had taken daily medication for constipation for many years.

The formula being given was a standard formula containing 1 Calorie per millilitre, and it was therefore decided to commence a fibre formula with increased water intake. Within a week Mary's stools were softer and her bowels were open three times per week.

Nausea and vomiting

Nausea and vomiting can be due to incorrect delivery, or too much formula being delivered too quickly. Nurses should slow down the rate and reconsider the amount being given.

Body position should be upright if possible, or at a 30-degree angle. The person should be left upright after feeding to allow for absorption of contents.

It can also be helpful to ensure that formula is at room temperature by allowing formula to stand for 30 minutes after removal from the refrigerator.

Reflux

Reflux and subsequent entry of gastric contents into the respiratory tract can cause irritation and predispose to an infection that can develop into aspiration pneumonia. An incorrect body position and/or too much formula too quickly can make reflux more likely to occur.

A feeding pump can be used to slow down the rate—thus achieving a more accurate and slower delivery. Checking gastric residuals before feeding might be indicated. Older people often eat small amounts more frequently and do not require the same volume. For those who are receiving palliative care, special consideration might have to be given to amounts and frequency of feeding.

A jejunostomy tube can be inserted into the jejunum, thus bypassing the stomach. In these circumstances, a feeding pump and continuous feeding will be required because large volumes are not tolerated by the jejunum.

Disengaged tube

A disengaged tube is caused by the tube being pulled out, the balloon bursting, or tube degradation. Because the tract closes within 1–2 hours (even in mature tracts), a spare tube should be available for immediate reinsertion.

If a suitably qualified person is not available to replace the gastrostomy tube, the person must go to a hospital to have a replacement tube inserted. Nurses should cover the tube site with a small gauze dressing and take the old tube with the person to the hospital. This assists with identification of the type and size of tube required.

Psychological adjustment

Eating is a social experience, and the prospect of never being able to eat or drink again is a very difficult situation to accept for both the person involved and for his or her family. It can become a very isolating experience. The nurse can be supportive and sympathetic, but expert psychological help might be necessary.

'The prospect of never being able to eat or drink again is a very difficult situation to accept.'

How long does the tube last?

PEG tube

A polyurethane PEG tube lasts for 5–6 years, and is a good choice for older people. A silicone PEG tube lasts for only 1–2 years. The silicone material can be invaded by a fungus, which gives the tube a pitted and lumpy look. Eventually, the internal lumen will collapse, and the tube has to be changed.

It is important to note whether the tube is for endoscopic or non-endoscopic removal. If the tube has a rigid internal disc it is necessary to return to hospital for an endoscopic removal. If the tube has a soft, inverted, internal bumper it can be removed externally through the stoma site at the bedside.

Balloon tube and low-profile balloon device

The replaceable balloon tube lasts for 3–10 months, depending on gastric acidity, medication, and tube movement. It is advisable to have a spare tube available for replacement if needed.

Low-profile stomate or button device

These devices have a dome-shaped or mushroom-shaped internal bumper, and can last for 1–2 years. They are removed by external traction and are very difficult for the recipient to remove accidentally.

Not being able to eat and drink means that important aspects of quality of life have been denied tube-fed people, but a cup of tea or a glass of wine passed down the tube, along with some of the tea or wine painted on the tongue, can help to break the tedium. Depending on the person's condition, a little oral diet (in the form of chewing of favourite foods and then spitting them out) might be acceptable. Chewing sugarless gum can also be helpful.

Conclusion

For more than twenty years, the percutaneous endoscopic approach to gastrostomy placement has gained widespread acceptance because of its ease and safety in placement. Health professionals have become very proactive in considering enteral feeding as an appropriate long-term method of feeding.

The increasing use of enteral nutrition in hospitals and residential aged care has led to an expanded role for gastroenterologists, dietitians, stomal therapists, and community health carers. Nurses have a vital role to play in the physical and psychological support of those in their care who are unable to take nutrition orally.

Chapter 8

Incontinence

Keren Day

Introduction

Being continent is a complex and important human skill. Continence can be defined as the ability to store and pass urine and faeces in socially acceptable places and times. It is one of the first skills of independent living learned as infants. For this reason, being incontinent is a difficult experience for a person because it involves the loss of this early skill. Dealing with incontinence is further complicated by its associations with body excrement, bacteria and other microorganisms, and strict social rules and taboos (Lawler 1991). It is therefore not surprising that incontinence is often hidden, rarely discussed, and generally not handled well by healthcare professionals or the community in general.

Incontinence is frequently encountered by nurses and personal carers, particularly in Care Homes. Cleaning up the mess and keeping a person comfortable is certainly an important part of the nurses' and carers' roles. However, it is also important to understand what incontinence is, who it affects, why it happens, and what can be done about it. It is possible to improve, and even cure, a person's incontinence problem. In some cases, incontinence can be prevented.

Effective nursing care involves more than keeping someone clean, dry, and comfortable. In dealing with incontinence, nurses must acknowledge that it is a problem that affects people physically, psychologically, and socially. Care for people who live with incontinence must therefore incorporate all of these elements. Although incontinence is not life-threatening, it is a problem that deeply affects people's quality of life.

> 'Effective nursing care involves more than keeping someone clean, dry, and comfortable . . . incontinence affects people physically, psychologically, and socially.'

Definitions

An internationally accepted definition of urinary incontinence is 'the involuntary loss of urine which is objectively demonstrable and a social or hygiene problem' (Abrams et al. 2002, p. 1080). Faecal incontinence can be defined as the involuntary or inappropriate passage of faeces (Norton et al. 2002).

Prevalence

Urinary incontinence is a problem that extends across the entire population to affect men, women, and children of all ages. However, those most likely to experience incontinence are children, pregnant women, menopausal women, people with disabilities, older people, and people in institutional care.

In assessing risk of incontinence, some influential predisposing factors have been recognised. Frail older people in Care Homes have many of these risk factors—including parity (number of births), ageing, constipation, urinary tract infections, impaired mobility, impaired cognition, and institutionalisation (Button et al. 1998).

There is some variation in the reported incidence of incontinence. This is because of differences in how incontinence is defined, the population groups surveyed, and the methods used for surveys (Mohide 1992). However, it is clear that the incidence of incontinence increases with age, and varies with different care settings. Women experience urinary incontinence at least twice as often as men, although this gender difference evens out in older people (Hunskaar et al. 1999). In people aged between 15 and 64 years of age, 1.5–5% suffer from urinary incontinence. Between 11% and 35% of people who are older than 60 and still living in the community are incontinent of urine (Roberts et al. 1999). At least 50% of elderly people in institutionalised care are incontinent of urine (AHCPR 1996; Ouslander & Schnelle 1995).

> 'At least 50% of elderly people in institutionalised care are incontinent of urine.'

Less research has been conducted on the problem of faecal incontinence. However, this is changing, and faecal incontinence is increasingly a focus of continence management. Faecal incontinence is not as common as urinary incontinence, and is experienced by 1–2% of the general population (Norton 1997). Like urinary incontinence, faecal incontinence is more common in women than in men in the younger age groups. However, the incidence increases with age and institutionalisation, and there is therefore a smaller difference in prevalence between men and women in a Care Home population (Norton et al. 2002). About 10% of older people living in the community are faecally incontinent. However up to 35% of older people in residential care experience this problem (Campbell, Reinken & McCosh 1985; Roberts et al. 1999).

There is a link between urinary and faecal incontinence. People with one type of incontinence are more likely to experience the other (Roberts et al. 1999).

Attitudes to incontinence

Of all people who experience incontinence, very few seek help for their problem. This reluctance to seek assistance is reinforced by many myths and false beliefs. It is commonly believed that incontinence is an inevitable part of childbirth or growing old, and that there is no hope of cure or improvement. Some people avoid disclosure, fearing that they will be treated negatively. Indeed, many people successfully hide the problem for years.

Incontinence, particularly faecal incontinence, is commonly believed to be a primary reason for placement in residential care. However, the issue is complex. In some cases, an incontinence problem might have been present for many years, but becomes recognised only after that person has been admitted to residential care. Incontinence does, however, substantially increase the need for hospitalisation and admission to residential care (Thom, Haan & Van den Eeden 1997).

Just as people with incontinence are reluctant to talk about the problem, health professionals and carers are also sometimes reluctant to discuss it. Nurses should create opportunities for people to disclose incontinence problems. To achieve this, nurses need to be comfortable with the issue themselves, have a positive attitude, be willing to ask the appropriate questions, and know what to do when a person does admit to being incontinent.

> 'Nurses should create opportunities for people to disclose incontinence problems.'

Incontinence in residential care

Incontinence is a major care need in residential aged care because older people in long-term institutional care are generally frailer, have more medical conditions, and are more dependent than their counterparts in the general population.

The myth that incontinence is an inevitable part of ageing is commonly believed by older residents themselves (Robinson 2000), as well as by those who care for them (Yu et al. 1991). This acceptance of incontinence as inevitable can mean that residents and staff are not open to strategies that are curative. Rather, strategies become aimed at simply concealing and coping with the incontinence (Robinson 2000). A 'mop-up' or containment approach to care can result. Some nurses believe that an 'across-the-board', 2-hourly toileting program and use of pads is the only solution. Continence programs that are not based on individual assessment waste nursing time and money, and require rethinking (Jilek 1993).

> 'The myth that incontinence is an inevitable part of ageing is commonly believed by elderly residents themselves, as well as by those who care for them.'

Incontinence increases the cost of residential care—including extra nursing time, extra supplies, and extra cleaning and laundry costs. In addition, incontinence predisposes residents to skin breakdown, urinary tract infections, and greater risk of falls, and can adversely affect residents psychologically and socially.

The cost is also carried by staff. Incontinence contributes to staff stress by increasing frustration and by being an uncomfortable and unpleasant problem to deal with. This is reflected in absenteeism and decreased staff retention in residential care (Yu et al. 1991).

Types and causes of incontinence

To be continent a person needs to be:

▶ aware of the need to pass urine or a bowel motion;
▶ able to get to the toilet;
▶ able to store the urine or the bowel motion before reaching
  the toilet;
▶ able to undress and get onto the toilet in time;
▶ able to empty the bladder or rectum (lower bowel) on cue once on
  or at the toilet; and
▶ able to complete the process by wiping, redressing, and so on.

The various causes of urinary incontinence can be categorised as follows
(Norton 1996a):

▶ physiological bladder dysfunction (an unstable bladder or stress
  incontinence);
▶ factors influencing bladder function (urinary tract infection, faecal
  impaction, or drugs); and
▶ factors affecting the ability to cope with the bladder (immobility, the
  environment, mental function, and inadequate patient care).

Table 8.1 (below) shows some common causes of incontinence.

Table 8.1 Causes of incontinence

Causes	Common examples
Loose stools or diarrhoea	inflammatory bowel disease, bowel infection, medicines, inadequate dietary fibre intake
Faecal impaction or loading	due to institutionalisation, immobility, poor diet and fluid intake, medicines
Ano-rectal problem	surgery to area anal sphincter or pelvic floor damage haemorrhoids, rectal prolapse, fistula
Neurological disease and other disabilities	spinal cord injury, multiple sclerosis, spina bifida, Parkinson's disease
Impaired cognition	dementia
Environmental barriers	poor toilet facilities and inadequate care
Idiopathic	unknown cause possible psychological factors

Authors' creation

Urinary incontinence can be categorised into four main types:

- urge incontinence;
- stress incontinence;
- overflow incontinence; and
- functional incontinence.

Urge incontinence is the involuntary passing of urine associated with a strong desire to void. People with urge incontinence typically have urinary urgency and frequency, and often say that they can't 'hold on' long enough to get to the toilet.

Stress incontinence is the involuntary passing of urine resulting from an increase in abdominal pressure (for example, during coughing, sneezing, or laughing). The bladder itself is quite relaxed and is not contracting. Women frequently experience stress incontinence, which is usually experienced as small amounts of leakage while coughing, laughing, lifting, or jumping.

Types of urinary incontinence

Urinary incontinence can be divided into the following categories.

Urge incontinence

Urge incontinence is the involuntary passing of urine associated with a strong desire to void.

Stress incontinence

Stress incontinence is the involuntary passing of urine resulting from an increase in abdominal pressure (for example, during coughing, sneezing, or laughing).

Overflow incontinence

Overflow incontinence occurs when the bladder is unable to empty normally, and fills up until it overflows.

Functional incontinence

Functional incontinence results from factors affecting the person's ability to cope with elimination, rather than from a problem with bladder function itself.

Overflow incontinence occurs when the bladder is unable to empty normally, and fills up until it overflows. This might be because the bladder muscle (the detrusor) is unable to contract effectively to expel the urine, or because there is an obstruction in the bladder outlet through which urine cannot pass. Typical symptoms include hesitancy when starting to void, poor or interupted urinary stream, frequency, having to urinate more often than normal overnight (nocturia), and not feeling completely empty at the end of a void.

Functional incontinence results from factors affecting the person's ability to cope with elimination, rather than from a problem with bladder function itself.

Factors such as reduced mobility, confusion, or obstacles in the environment are causes of this type of incontinence.

The mechanisms that cause each of these types of incontinence are different and there can be more than one type of incontinence present in a person. The management strategies that are used are specific to the type of problem, and thorough individual assessment is therefore required.

> 'The management strategies that are used are specific to the type of problem, and thorough individual assessment is therefore required.'

Assessment and management

In the UK, a full continence assessment should be carried out by a registered nurse before continence products are prescribed for a Care Home resident. The NHS is then responsible for provision of the continence products, if required. The causes of incontinence must always be investigated, and, where possible, treated.

A thorough assessment identifies the factors that are affecting the person's ability to be continent, and enables a diagnosis of the type of incontinence to be made. This allows an approriate plan of management to be developed.

A plethora of continence assessment tools and forms has been developed to assist in answering these questions. Whatever form, tool, or framework is used, it should include:

- the person's perception of the problem;
- functional assessment of the person's capabilities (including mobility, dexterity, mental status, and personal care needs);
- social situation;
- medical history (including surgical, obstetric, gynaecological, and urological histories);
- current medications (both prescribed and unprescribed medications, and how they are actually taken);
- dietary and fluid intake;
- bowel status (including any current bowel management used); and
- bladder status (the specifics of the problem, such as how often the person is wet, extent of wetness, how many times the person voids, characteristics of the urinary stream, and so on).

Once the continence assessment has been completed, management can be planned and implemented. The goal of incontinence management is a person's quality of life—not simply keeping him or her dry. Even though some residents remain incontinent, their problems can be managed in a way that maintains their comfort and dignity, so that their incontinence is not obvious to others and the person does not need to refrain from any activity in which he or she wishes to participate.

> 'The goal of incontinence management is a person's quality of life—not simply keeping him or her dry.'

It is helpful to view the process of continence assessment and management as having three levels:

◗ ensuring that the basic needs for continence are in place
◗ screening for, and treating, common reversible causes of incontinence; and
◗ assessing and managing persistent incontinence.

Each of these is discussed below.

Level 1: Basic needs for continence

It is important to assess the basic factors that affect a person's ability to maintain continence. When these 'basics' are in place, some incontinence can be cured. Perhaps more importantly, some incontinence can be *prevented*. The foundations for healthy bladder function include:

◗ adequate fluid intake;
◗ healthy toileting habits; and
◗ appropriate bowel patterns.

Adequate fluid intake

A daily fluid intake of approximately 6–8 glasses (1.5–2.0 litres) should be maintained unless otherwise advised by a doctor. Fluid should always be available and accessible, taking into account particular likes and dislikes. Offering small, frequent drinks is more effective than occasional larger volumes when attempting to increase fluid intake.

Caffeine consumption (for example, tea, coffee, and cola drinks) should be limited because caffeine is a bladder irritant that increases the sense of urgency. It is also a diuretic. Alcohol should also be limited because of its diuretic effect. In place of caffeinated and alcoholic drinks, nurses can provide decaffeinated fluids and herbal alternatives.

Healthy toileting habits

Nurses can assist people to maintain healthy toileting habits, which help to prevent and improve bladder problems. These habits include not going to the toilet 'just in case'. Rather, people should be encouraged to go the toilet in response to feeling the urge to void. They should also be allowed adequate time and privacy at the toilet, thus ensuring that the void is finished properly and that the bladder is empty. Nurses should also ensure that people visit the toilet an appropriate number of times each day, based on the understanding that it is normal to void between four to six times per 24 hours, including a maximum of once or twice overnight. The volume passed should be about 300–500 millilitres each time.

Nurses can also promote the best positioning for toileting. The position that best promotes effective bladder and bowel emptying is squatting. Western-style toilets do not accommodate this position, but it is possible for a person to sit with feet slightly elevated on a small step stool, leaning forward, with legs slightly apart, and elbows resting on knees. This enables the best-possible pelvic position, and aligns the bladder and bowel with their outlets so that gravity assists evacuation. Straining to empty the bladder or the bowel should be discouraged because this can weaken the muscles of the pelvic floor.

Monitoring a resident's toileting habits can be difficult, especially in a large Care Home. The best way to get an accurate picture of a resident's bladder and bowel status is to complete a continence chart that documents a person's toileting and incontinence pattern over a period of three days to a week. Bladder charts can take many forms, and some are extremely complex. All charts need to provide such basic information as frequency of voiding, frequency of incontinent episodes, and voided volumes. There should also be a place for comment or explanation.

Appropriate bowel patterns

Maintaining regular bowel function is an important part of preventing both urinary and faecal incontinence. Constipation is one of the most common causes of urinary and faecal incontinence in older people. To prevent constipation, or to treat mild forms of constipation, nurses should ensure that the basic foundations for maintenance of a satisfactory bowel pattern are in place. These include eating a high-fibre diet (and eating enough in general), an adequate fluid intake, daily gentle exercise, and avoidance of constipating drugs and foods.

The best-possible positioning on the toilet (see above) promotes effective emptying of the bowel.

Timing toileting to take greatest advantage of the gastro-colic reflex (which occurs within 30 minutes after meals) is a useful strategy in preventing both constipation and faecal incontinence.

Assessment and management of incontinence

This section of the chapter discusses assessment and management of incontinence under the following headings:

Level 1: Basic needs for continence
- adequate fluid intake;
- healthy toileting habits; and
- appropriate bowel patterns.

Level 2: Common reversible causes of incontinence
- medications;
- impaired mobility;
- impaired cognition;
- environmental problems;
- urinary tract infection; and
- constipation and impaction of faeces.

Level 3: Assessment and management of persistent incontinence
- bladder dysfunction;
- bowel dysfunction; and
- continence products.

Level 2: Common reversible causes of incontinence

If the basic foundations for continence are in place, and the problem persists, the next step is to check for some of the common causes of incontinence that are potentially reversible. These reversible causes of incontinence include:

- medications;
- impaired mobility;
- impaired cognition;
- environmental problems;
- urinary tract infection; and
- constipation and impaction of faeces.

Medications

A review of medicines taken by a person might reveal some commonly prescribed medications that can contribute to urinary or faecal incontinence. These include drugs that can have a constipating effect—such as iron tablets, some antidepressants, most analgesics, and some diuretics.

Bladder emptying can be impaired by drugs that have an anticholinergic action, such as some antidepressants.

Prescribed sedatives should also be part of any review of medications.

Impaired mobility

Reduced mobility can delay or prevent a person from getting to the toilet, and can be a primary cause or a contributing factor to incontinence. The condition causing the immobility might be treatable, or might be capable of being improved through rehabilitation or use of walking aids. For example, a person with severe arthritis might experience less incontinence if better pain management is implemented or if a walking frame is provided. A referral to an appropriate medical or allied health professional might achieve improved function.

Nurses should also ensure that residents are using mobility aids appropriately. There are multiple benefits of improving mobility and increasing activity for residents. Improvement in incontinence problems is one such significant benefit.

Impaired cognition

Impaired cognitive function can contribute to the development of incontinence in a variety of ways. Impaired memory might result in a resident forgetting the toilet location, or being highly distractable and unable to focus on the task of getting to the toilet. Inhibition might be affected, which can result in inappropriate voiding. Cognitive impairment might also mean that a person is unable to identify the sensation of a full bladder, or know what to do about it, despite feeling restless or agitated.

> 'A person might be unable to identify the sensation of a full bladder, or know what to do about it.'

These various cognitive problems require different management strategies to achieve continence. A medical assessment might be indicated, particularly if the confusion or changes have occurred quickly, in which case the underlying cause might be treatable.

Management strategies include:

- prompts (in the form of appropriate signage, verbal cues, and directions from staff);
- nurses toileting a person in response to a signal from them (for example, pacing or plucking at trousers); and
- nurses toileting people at timed intervals (based on a continence assessment chart).

Prompted voiding, using a combination of caregiver prompts and positive reinforcement, is one of the most effective toileting strategies for elderly people with cognitive impairment. However, one of the greatest barriers to the effectiveness of any toileting strategy is a lack of staff adherence to the toileting schedule.

Environmental problems

Environmental barriers to continence include lack of privacy, difficulty opening toilet doors, the height of the toilet seat, lack of space to manoeuvre in the toilet, steps, lack of available staff to assist a frail older person to the toilet, and even staff attitudes. Some of these barriers can be removed or overcome, whereas others must be accommodated in the management plan. Often such interventions are common sense, but all environmental factors are nevertheless vitally important considerations in the development of a management plan.

Urinary tract infection

Every person with urinary incontinence should have a routine urine analysis early in the assessment process to exclude a urinary tract infection (UTI). A urinalysis 'dip stick' positive to nitrite indicates whether further laboratory testing is required. Signs and symptoms such as burning or discomfort while passing urine, cloudy and offensive smelling urine, and an increased frequency indicate that a UTI is present. However, an infection might not be symptomatic. More general symptoms, such as increased confusion and fever, can be the only indications of a UTI in an elderly person.

> 'Every person with urinary incontinence should have a routine urine analysis early in the assessment process.'

Management strategies that can support medical treatment of a UTI include encouraging extra fluids (unless otherwise contraindicated), especially fluids that can make the urine more alkaline. Other supportive strategies include wearing nonrestrictive pants and clothing, eliminating the use of talcum powder and perfumed soap, and the use (and frequent changing) of quality continence products.

Constipation and impaction of faeces

Constipation and impaction can cause both urinary and faecal incontinence. If there is no improvement once the basics of optimal bowel care are in place, further assessment is required. A period of bowel charting recording the frequency, timing, and characteristics of bowel motions is advisable. It is helpful to chart fluid and dietary input at the same time as charting bowel pattern.

Constipation can have a variety of causes. Involving a doctor is often advisable because an abdominal and rectal examination, and a plain abdominal x-ray, can assist in determining the severity and extent of the problem. A review of medications that have constipating side-effects is also required.

Laxatives are frequently used in residential care—often inappropriately and excessively (Norton et al. 2002). They have many different ways of acting and it is important that the right agent is used. They must be treated with the same caution with which all drugs should be used. Laxatives should be used after a thorough bowel assessment has taken place and after all other non-pharmacological strategies have been attempted.

> 'Laxatives are frequently used in residential care—often inappropriately and excessively.'

Level 3: Assessment and management of persistent incontinence

When a problem does not respond to initial efforts of putting the basic foundations for continence in place (Level 1 management, as outlined above) or to screening and treatment for the known common causes of incontinence (Level 2 management above), specialist continence assessment is required. A referral to a continence specialist or service might be appropriate.

Such an assessment will include consideration of the following:

▶ bladder dysfunction;
▶ bowel dysfunction; and
▶ continence products.

Each of these is considered below.

Bladder dysfunction

Assessing a person for specific bladder dysfunction (such as an unstable bladder or an undercontractile bladder) includes taking a more detailed history. A continence-management plan based on a specific diagnosis can then be developed in consultation with nurses who carry out the daily care.

Management might include bladder retraining, a specific toileting regimen, a pelvic-muscle rehabilitation program, and use of medications.

Medication, such as an anticholinergic drug to treat an unstable bladder, might be considered for carefully selected elderly residents (Ouslander & Schnelle 1995; Ouslander et al. 2001). However, a decision to prescribe any medication in frail older people, many of whom take a variety of other drugs, must be made with great care because of the potential complications and interactions.

Management might also include the use of catheterisation (both intermittent and indwelling), although this is generally a management option used as a last resort. Management at night also needs to be individualised to minimise interuption to sleep. It should be based on skin-care needs, rather than the convenience of staffing routines.

> 'Management at night should be based on skin-care needs, rather than the convenience of staffing routines.'

Bowel dysfunction

Bowel dysfunction—such as an impaired anal sphincter or constipation and impaction not responsive to earlier strategies—involves a more detailed assessment. A specialist medical opinion might be appropriate, and this might involve further testing—such as gastric transit times and anal pressure (manometry) studies. An assessment of the biodynamics of bowel evacuation might be part of the assessment of bowel dysfunction, and this involves a detailed observation of position and the sequencing and use of muscle groups that need to coordinate for complete evacuation of the bowel.

Management might also include further dietary manipulation, the use of appropriate medications, and muscle re-education. Surgical options might be explored as appropriate treatment for some people. Re-education using biofeedback might be required with respect to positioning and use of the appropriate muscle groups during bowel evacuation (Norton 1997).

Continence products

It is sometimes not possible to resolve the incontinence of many older people in residential care. The appropriate use of continence products is one way of achieving quality of life.

Because continence products for Care Home residents are supplied by the NHS, products may be specified by the local continence service. This follows an assessment of each resident, which may be carried out when the NHS contribution to nursing care is determined. A NHS employed nurse undertakes these assessments, in consultation with the Care Home staff. If residents or their carers wish to purchase continence products privately, they may do so. Continence advisors are also available to provide additional specialist advice if required.

Some principles in selecting an appropriate continence product are outlined in the Box below.

Selecting a continence product

As in all other aspects of continence management, the selection of continence products must be based on an individual assessment. A person might need to use a number of different types of products as their condition and activities change.

In choosing the right product for a person, it is important to consider the following factors:

- gender;
- physical size and shape of the person;
- amount and character of the incontinence (for example, large volumes in gushes);
- lifestyle and activities;
- clothing;
- independence with use/application, and toileting;
- laundry, storage, and disposal facilities;
- finances;
- availability of supply; and
- personal likes and dislikes.

The large range of continence products available include:

- disposable pads and pants/diapers for both urinary and faecal incontinence;
- washable pads and pants;
- condom drainage (also known as penile sheaths);
- absorbent bed and chair pads;
- intermittent and indwelling urinary catheters;
- faecal collectors and anal plugs; and
- bladder neck support devices and urethral plugs.

Information about the range of products available can be obtained through a local continence service or directly through companies and suppliers. The Internet is another source of information, although it is important to analyse information critically because commercial interests influence the way information is presented.

Conclusion

Urinary and faecal incontinence present enormous challenges for both sufferers and carers. They are multifaceted problems that affect people on physical, psychological, and social levels. Much more can be done than simply cleaning up messes, and changing beds and pads.

Effective continence care begins with ensuring that the basic foundations for continence are in place for every older person in residential care. This includes screening for, and dealing with, the common reversible causes of incontinence Specialist continence assessment and management might be required.

It is not realistic to aim to achieve 'dryness' for all older residents. However, it is possible to improve the well-being and quality of life of older incontinent people through increased staff knowledge and improved attitudes, reduction in the number of episodes of incontinence, and better management and containment of persistent incontinence.

> 'It is not realistic to aim to achieve 'dryness' for all, but it is possible to improve well-being and quality of life.'

Chapter 9

Falls

Keith Hill, Catherine Barrett, Robyn Smith, and Melissa Lindeman

Introduction

Falls among older people are common, with one in three people aged over 65 experiencing one or more falls during a 12-month period. The rate of falls is even higher in residential aged-care facilities, where up to 60% of residents fall in a 12-month period (Tinetti 1987). Serious injuries related to falls have been reported to occur in 9% of residents in Care Homes, with the most common serious injuries being hip fractures (38%), other fractures (30%), and lacerations (30%) (Thapa et al. 1996). Hip fractures, which are one of the most catastrophic injuries sustained following a fall, are ten times more likely following a fall in older people in Care Homes than those living in private homes (Butler et al. 1996). Many falls, although they might cause no injury or minimal injury, can have a marked effect on other areas—including loss of confidence in walking and reduced participation in regular activities. These factors can increase an older person's risk of falling in the future.

Preventable falls

Because falls are common in Care Homes there can be a perception among some staff members, residents, and family members that falls are inevitable, and that nothing can be done to prevent them. Recent developments in research and practice indicate that a range of actions can be effective in reducing falls and falls-related injuries among older people, including those in Care Homes (Hill et al. 2000a).

> 'A range of actions can be effective in reducing falls and falls-related injuries among older people.'

Data collection

An important first step in dealing with falls is to establish the magnitude of the problem within a particular Care Home setting, and to identify common circumstances relating to falls and falls injuries. There are often distinctive characteristics about each setting (for example, layout, floor surfaces, lighting), staffing mix, and resident profile (for example, age, mobility, proportion with cognitive impairment) that can influence the incidence and consequences of falls. A standardised falls incident report (see Figure 9.1, page 109) is useful in documenting information about falls. Intermittent review of such reports can indicate patterns of falls events, and these can lead to a refinement of care plans to reduce the risk of future falls. Falls incident data are being increasingly computerised, and this provides opportunities for trend analysis and feedback to staff.

Common circumstances or activities associated with falls in Care Homes include (Lipsitz et al. 1991):

- walking (53%);
- posture change (for example, standing up from a chair) (50%);
- getting out of bed (31%); and
- bathroom visit (13%).

The circumstances of falls resulting in injuries among older people in Care Homes have been shown to differ between ambulatory and non-ambulatory residents. Among non-ambulatory people, falls that cause injury are significantly more common in certain circumstances. These include (Thapa et al. 1996):

- during the day (7 am to 11 pm);
- from chair or bed level;

Falls Incident Report

Resident's name:

| Date of fall: | Time of fall: |

Name of witness(es):

Brief description of the fall:

Activity at time of fall: ◯ walking   ◯ getting in or out of chair or bed   ◯ other

Place where fall occurred: ◯ bedroom   ◯ bathroom   ◯ common room
◯ toilet   ◯ outside   ◯ dining room   ◯ other

Fell from: ◯ bed   ◯ chair   ◯ wheelchair   ◯ commode   ◯ toilet
◯ other   ◯ not applicable

Was the resident using a walking aid at time of incident?

Any environmental hazards identified:

Were there risk factors identified before the fall (in terms of the Falls Risk Assessment and Management Form)?

Is it clear how the fall might have been prevented?

Immediate impact of fall: ◯ no injury   ◯ bruising (where?) ....
◯ pain (where?) .... ◯ laceration/skin tear (where?) ....
◯ possible fracture (where?) ....

Nursing interventions: ◯ transfer to hospital   ◯ attend first aid treatments
◯ refer to general practitioner for immediate review
◯ refer to general practitioner on next visit
◯ alteration to medications   ◯ alteration to nursing care
◯ alteration to environment   ◯ discuss fall with patient
◯ discuss fall with family

Date to be reviewed:

Signature of staff member: **Date:**

Figure 9.1 Falls incident report form
Shanley (1998); © Commonwealth of Australia, published with permission

▶ while sitting or transferring; and
▶ in the presence of equipment (for example, wheelchair, commode, shower chair).

Other factors commonly associated with an increased risk of fall-related injuries include the use of restraints (Neufeld et al. 1999; van Leeuwen et al. 2001), osteoporosis, and osteomalacia.

Extrinsic and intrinsic risk factors

Risk factors for falls can be categorised as *extrinsic* (related to the environment or a high-risk activity being undertaken) or *intrinsic* (related to the ageing process or the influence of disease on the systems involved in balance). Examples of extrinsic and intrinsic risk factors for older people in residential care settings are listed in Table 9.1 (below). This table also identifies potential actions that might help with the management of each factor.

'Any management plan to reduce falls usually draws on a range of strategies.'

In the majority of cases, falls are multifactorial in nature and often involve a combination of extrinsic and intrinsic risk factors. Any management plan to reduce falls usually draws on a range of strategies.

Table 9.1 Falls and falls injury risk factors

Falls risk factors	Things to look for	Management options	Issues to consider
Intrinsic factors (falls)			
History of previous falls	review circumstances of falls; look for common themes for that individual	undertake assessment of falls risk factors and introduce appropriate management options	need to involve GP, physiotherapist, OT, or other staff and carers
Leg weakness	difficulty standing up from chair	refer to physiotherapist for assessment and strengthening exercises	program of exercises for staff or family to supervise

(Continued)

Table 9.1 Falls and falls injury risk factors *(Continued)*

Falls risk factors	Things to look for	Management options	Issues to consider
Intrinsic factors (falls)			
Balance problems and impaired walking	unsteady or veering during transfers and walking	refer to physiotherapist for assessment and balance exercises; consider use of walking aid	program of exercises for staff or family to supervise; physiotherapist can identify most appropriate walking aid, correct height, and instruct resident on correct use; residents often need repeated practice to learn to use a walking aid correctly
Functional impairments	difficulty with bed mobility, transfers, dressing, other personal activities of daily living	refer to OT for assessment re provision of aids and appliance or retraining; refer to physiotherapist for assessment and exercise	correct chair heights, rail heights and aids can improve residents' independence
Visual problems	hesitant gait, bumping into furniture, trips	ensure regular eye checks (at least every 2 years)	bifocals can be problematic on stairs or kerbs
Postural hypotension	unsteady or giddy when first stands up; can also be a problem soon after eating	review with GP; encourage resident to stand up slowly, and wait a short time before walking; might benefit from pressure stockings	medications review
Cognitive problems; dementia	poor planning, judgment, monitoring safety	review with GP	some patients benefit from cognitive-enhancing medications

(Continued)

Table 9.1 Falls and falls injury risk factors *(Continued)*

Falls risk factors	Things to look for	Management options	Issues to consider
Intrinsic factors (falls)			
Cognitive problems; dementia (cont.)	poor ability to follow instructions (e.g., using walking aid) or difficulty learning	increased surveillance (position of room, bed or chair alarms); review by physiotherapist re most appropriate walking aid, and whether resident will be able to use it safely; review by OT to consider training or compensatory strategies	might benefit from regular practice and reminders to use walking aid appropriately; others might find the walking aid 'gets in the way'
Medications (sedatives, anti-depressants, hypnotics)	any problems (e.g., unsteadiness or dizziness) soon after a change in medication	discuss medication issues with GP	some medications (e.g., benzodia-zepines) require gradual weaning if used for some time
	falls at night	review night-time medication use; use of commode at night	
More than 4 medications	review medication chart	discuss medication issues with GP; consider referral to geriatrician	
Chronic medical conditions (such as stroke, Parkinson's disease, arthritis)	these conditions often affect balance and mobility; sensation and perception can be altered; walking and balance performance often worsens over time	intermittent review by physiotherapist or OT with implementation of exercise program and appropriate aids	consider referral for assessment if there is a change in mobility or functional status or an increase in falls

(Continued)

Table 9.1 Falls and falls injury risk factors *(Continued)*

Falls risk factors	Things to look for	Management options	Issues to consider
Intrinsic factors (falls)			
Acute health problems (such as urinary tract infection, pneumonia, delirium)	rapid change or deterioration in function; often a short-term increase in unsteadiness and falls risk	urgent review by GP; acute medical care	short period of rehabilitation can be beneficial to restore function once acute problem is treated
Intrinsic factors (falls injuries)			
Osteoporosis (low bone density)	history of fractures; family history of osteoporosis; low bone density identified by bone scan	vitamin D and calcium supplementation; hip protectors	GP or dietitian review; different types of hip protectors available; problems associated with low compliance of residents with wearing hip protectors
Osteomalacia (low vitamin D)	vitamin D levels	nutritional assessment; vitamin D and calcium supplementation; sunlight exposure	
Extrinsic factors (falls and injuries)			
Relocation between settings	disorientation in new setting; increased confusion	take time to provide adequate orientation to new setting (repeat frequently if necessary)	family involvement

(Continued)

Table 9.1 Falls and falls injury risk factors *(Continued)*

Falls risk factors	Things to look for	Management options	Issues to consider
Extrinsic factors (falls and injuries)			
Environmental hazards	environmental hazards observed in any falls or near falls, no matter how minor they seem; common sites for falls (e.g., places where more than one resident experiences falls)	staff should perform environmental safety audits frequently; refer for an OT assessment to assess the resident's abilities in the context of the environment and make specific recommendations for the resident	review of the facility and surrounding environment, considering needs of all residents, staff, and visitors
Poor footwear	ill-fitting footwear; high heels inappropriate for anyone with balance problems; badly worn footwear (e.g., heels worn down on outside of shoe)	encourage use of safe, well-fitting footwear (discuss with family re need to purchase new shoes); refer for podiatry assessment	most appropriate shoes are low-heeled, lace-up, firm-fitting shoes with non-slip sole; slippers generally considered unsafe footwear

Authors' creation

Falls risk-assessment tool

A systematic approach to identifying falls risk factors is one of the most effective approaches to falls prevention in Care Homes. A structured assessment targeting environmental and personal safety, wheelchair use, psychotropic drug use, and transferring and ambulation can produce a significant reduction in recurrent falls and a reduction in falls-related injuries (Ray et al. 1997).

Important considerations when implementing a falls risk assessment include the following.

▶ *When should the falls risk assessment be completed?* Ideally falls risk assessments should be completed on admission to a facility, at regular intervals (for example, 6-monthly), or when there is change in function or an acute event (such as pneumonia, delirium, or a fall).

▶ *Who should complete the falls risk assessment and develop the appropriate care plan?* In many cases, nursing staff or physiotherapists are the most appropriate staff members to complete the falls risk assessment. Other team members (for example, occupational therapist, dietitian, general practitioner) can also make valuable contributions to assessment and planning.

▶ *What is the most appropriate falls risk-assessment tool to use?* There is no consensus about this. An example of a tool that has been used successfully in several residential care facilities is shown in Figure 9.2 (page 116).

Environmental falls hazard-assessment tool

There are many environmental hazards in residential aged-care facilities that have the potential to cause falls. Some common environmental hazards include:

▶ inadequate lighting;
▶ slippery bathroom surfaces;
▶ poor delineation between different floor surfaces;
▶ sun glare on floor surfaces;
▶ moss on outside footpaths;
▶ inadequate placement of rails in toilet or shower; residents then use inappropriate options for support (for example, pulling up on the toilet roll holder to stand);
▶ inadequate height chairs, poorly maintained chairs, insufficient number of chairs in long corridors; and
▶ wheeled equipment with inadequate brakes, or brakes not applied.

An example of an environmental falls risk hazard assessment is shown in Figure 9.3 (page 119). Regular and frequent environmental falls hazard assessments should be undertaken, and actions to minimise risks should be followed through.

The interaction between an individual resident and his or her environment can also be an important factor in determining whether a specific situation is safe or not. For example, one chair type or height might be appropriate for one resident in terms of ease of sit to stand, minimising effort, and decreasing a tendency to overbalance, but the same chair might be far too high for another resident. In more complex situations, a comprehensive assessment by an occupational therapist will identify the most appropriate actions to ensure the greatest safety for a resident within his or her environment.

Falls Risk Assessment and Management Form

Name of resident:

Problem or issue	Assessment	Yes or No	Management options (tick which ones you suggest)
Medications	• Does the person take 4 or more medications in total? or • Does the person take one or more psychotropics (tranquillisers, antidepressants or sedative/hypnotics)?		• Allocate to high-risk group • Review by GP to try to reduce medications or dosages
Acute illness	• Does the person have any sign of acute illness eg. altered behaviour, confusion, pain, malaise, fever, cough, urinary symptoms		• Review by GP to ensure appropriate treatment
Mental state	• Is the person confused and/or disoriented and/or wandering?		• Refer to GP to exclude treatable causes • Allocate to high-risk group
Ongoing medical conditions	• Does the person have: — CVA? — Parkinson's disease? — Osteoarthritis in knees/hips? — Dementia? — Postural hypotension? — Depression? — Dizziness?		• Allocate to high-risk group • Review by GP to ensure optimum treatment • Refer to physiotherapist for possible treatments
History of previous falls	• Has the person had: — one fall in past year which requires treatment or — more than two falls not requiring treatment in past year?		• Allocate to high-risk group (Continued)

Figure 9.2 Risk-assessment tool
Shanley (1998); © Commonwealth of Australia, published with permission

Falls Risk Assessment and Management Form *(Continued)*

Name of resident:

Problem or issue	Assessment	Yes or No	Management options (tick which ones you suggest)
Poor balance	• Is the person unsafe when asked to stand from chair, walk 3 metres, turn and return to chair independently (even with walking aid)?		• Allocate to high-risk group • Refer to GP for assessment • Refer to physiotherapist for assessment
Use of walking aids	• Does the person use or need aids to mobilise?		• Allocate to high-risk group • Assess use of aids according to guidelines in this manual • Refer to physiotherapist for specialist assessment and treatment
Bowel or bladder problems	• Does the person have urinary or faecal incontinence, or urgency during the day or night?		• Institute appropriate nursing care • Refer to GP for assessment • Allocate to high-risk group
Visual problems	• Does the person (while using their normal glasses) have problems reading headlines in the newspaper, making out figures on the TV or seeing objects alongside them?		• Refer to GP and ophthalmologist to exclude cataracts or other treatable disease and review glasses • Refer to optometrist for revision of existing glasses • Allocate to high-risk group if there is poor vision which cannot be corrected
Hearing problems	• Does the person have problems hearing you with normal speech?		• Refer to GP for checking of ears and hearing • Refer to audiologist for hearing aid assessment • Ensure hearing aids are working and being used correctly • Allocate to high-risk group if there is poor hearing which cannot be corrected *(Continued)*

Figure 9.2 Risk-assessment tool *(Continued)*

Shanley (1998); © Commonwealth of Australia, published with permission

Falls Risk Assessment and Management Form (*Continued*)
Name of resident:

Problem or issue	Assessment	Yes or No	Management options (tick which ones you suggest)
Feet problems	• Does the person have corns, ingrown toenails, ulcers, deformities or infection of the feet?		• Institute appropriate nursing care • Refer to podiatrist for treatment • Allocate to high-risk group if problems cannot be successfully treated
Footwear	• Does the person have unsafe footwear, according to guidelines in this manual		• Correct problems, according to guidelines in this manual

Signature of staff member: **Date:**

Figure 9.2 Risk-assessment tool
Shanley (1998); © Commonwealth of Australia, published with permission

Changing practice

Some educational strategies and approaches to communication are more likely to lead to practice change than others. The use of appropriate educational strategies and communication structures is more likely to produce sustainable changes in practice. Falls prevention should become part of the culture of the Care Home or ward, and part of the everyday responsibility of key staff in the multidisciplinary team. A culture of resident-centred care, in which all members of staff work together to meet the resident's needs is likely to be more effective in preventing falls and related injury on an ongoing basis than a culture in which there is limited communication between staff and a hierarchical structure with autocratic management. A responsive organisational culture will help to ensure sustainability of change.

> 'Falls prevention should become part of the culture . . . part of the everyday responsibility of staff in the multidisciplinary team.'

GENERAL ENVIRONMENTAL HAZARD CHECKLIST:
To be completed via general audit.

Flooring	Indoors		
	Non-slip surfaces	Yes	No
	Absence of raised edge	Yes	No
	Good condition	Yes	No
Circulation	Absence of clutter	Yes	No
	Adequate storage for equipment	Yes	No
	Adequate space for mobility aids	Yes	No
Visibility	Walls contrasting colour to floor	Yes	No
	Handrails contrasting colour to walls	Yes	No
	Rails contrasting colour to background	Yes	No
	Steps edges contrasting colour	Yes	No
	Absence of glare from windows	Yes	No
Lighting	Well-lit hallways and rooms (75 watts)	Yes	No
	Stairs well lit day and night?	Yes	No
Bathroom	Non-slip flooring	Yes	No
	Step-less shower base	Yes	No
	Room for seat near to shower	Yes	No
	Room for seat in shower	Yes	No
	Free of clutter (storage of equipment)	Yes	No
	Rail in shower / near toilet	Yes	No
	Lightweight door / easy to use	Yes	No
Bedroom	Adequate space for frame access	Yes	No
	Bedspreads clear from floor	Yes	No
	Call button within reach	Yes	No
Rails	Handgrips along walls in all areas	Yes	No
	Handrails on all steps	Yes	No
	Beside toilet	Yes	No
	In shower	Yes	No
Signs	Clear/Adequate signs throughout	Yes	No
Outdoors	Absence of potholes	Yes	No
	Even pathway	Yes	No
	Sufficient width for two people (inc. one using frame)	Yes	No
	No overhanging branches	Yes	No

(Continued)

Figure 9.3 Environmental hazard checklist

Falls Prevention Service, Peninsula Health Care Network (1999); published with permission

GENERAL ENVIRONMENTAL HAZARD CHECKLIST:

To be completed via general audit.

Outdoors			
	Paths clear of shrubs, bushes	Yes	No
	Regular removal/sweeping of leaves on paths	Yes	No
	Non-slip steps and step edges	Yes	No
	Steps in good condition	Yes	No
	Sufficient number of outdoor seats for regular rest	Yes	No
	Outdoor seating secure/sufficient height	Yes	No

ACTION/S REQUIRED: BY WHOM

Assessed by .... Date ....

Figure 9.3 Environmental hazard checklist
Falls Prevention Service, Peninsula Health Care Network (1999); published with permission

Communication

Effective communication is especially important. Attention should be given to how communication is managed *between* and *within* all the groups involved in care giving—registered nurses, healthcare assistants, ancillary staff (cleaners, food attendants, and so on), relatives, residents, volunteers, management, administrative staff, doctors, and allied health staff. The Box below presents some tips on effective communication.

Tips for effective communication

A range of practical strategies to promote communication can be adopted to facilitate practice change and development. These include (Lindeman et al. 2002):

- seeking ways to encourage communication and sharing of ideas between staff of all backgrounds and classifications;
- valuing the input of all staff whose work contributes to resident care;
- encouraging staff to develop ideas for practice change and being prepared to trial new initiatives;
- ensuring that there are regular opportunities for *all* staff to attend staff meetings, and encouraging discussion and learning;
- investigating ways of establishing mechanisms for direct care staff to regularly discuss individual resident needs

Education

The effectiveness of traditional lecture-style approaches to continuing professional education in health settings is limited (Davis & Thomson 1996), and it is therefore important to consider more contemporary methods that are based on sound adult-learning principles. A program of staff education, on its own, does not necessarily lead to a significant reduction in the rate of falls (Lieu et al. 1997), even though staff knowledge might increase following a traditional didactic presentation (Taylor & Morris 1999). It is apparent that education or training alone, without strategies to enable newly acquired knowledge to be translated into sustainable practice, will have limited effectiveness. The Box below presents some tips on effective methods of education.

> 'Education or training alone, without strategies to translate this into sustainable practice, will have limited effectiveness.'

Tips for effective methods of education

When planning education in residential aged care, consideration should be given to:

- all the groups involved in the facility—registered nurses, healthcare assistants, ancillary staff (cleaners, food attendants, and so on), relatives, residents, volunteers, management and administrative staff, general practitioners, allied health professionals, and others as considered appropriate;
- what each of these groups needs to know about falls and falls prevention;
- whether these groups have access to the information they need; and
- how these groups acquire and apply additional information to improve practice and reduce falls.

If workforce training is to be effective, the focus must be on changing the behaviour of the staff, rather than individual behaviour—because it is group behaviour that affects the health outcome for older people in these settings (Redman et al. 1999). Such behavioural change is facilitated if staff members are actively involved in problem-solving and decision-making, and if staff involvement in the identification of issues and actions is encouraged. Other helpful strategies include follow-up and support for staff members when they are back on the job following training sessions.

Learning opportunities should be presented in a variety of formats (Lindeman et al. 2000). Interactive learning and an experiential approach to staff training in a comprehensive falls-prevention program have been shown to be effective in a Care Home setting (Hill et al. 2002). These approaches provide staff members with the opportunity to apply knowledge as they learn.

Conclusion

Falls are common for older people in residential care, and these falls usually have multiple causes. A range of falls-prevention activities can reduce falls and injuries. However, to be effective and sustainable, falls-prevention practice should be integrated into standard assessments, care planning, environment audits, and ongoing clinical and facility management.

To achieve the goal of reduced falls and falls injuries, staff members, residents, family members, and carers need to work collaboratively to develop and implement the most appropriate mix of strategies for individual residents.

Chapter 10

Manual Handling and Mobility

Lynn Varcin-Coad

Introduction

Manual handling of people refers to any activity requiring the use of force or effort by a person to lift, carry, lower, push, pull, support, move, hold, or restrain another person. The mobility and manual handling of people is an important aspect of care of older people. It is also an integral part of occupational health-and-safety practice for both residents and staff.

There is a higher-than-average incidence of back pain among nursing staff (Videman et al. 1984; Worksafe Australia 1994), and this is related to the lifting and manual handling of patients (Garg et al. 1991). To minimise injury to nursing staff, the Royal College of Nursing in the United Kingdom initiated guidelines for safer manual handling. The suggested policy stated (RCN 1996):

> 'Mobility and manual handling is an important aspect of aged care and occupational health and safety.'

. . . the manual lifting of patients is eliminated in all but exceptional or life threatening situations . . . patients are encouraged to assist in their own transfers, and handling aids must be used whenever they can help to reduce risk, if this is not contrary to a patient's needs.

This policy required a risk-management approach, constant reassessment of patient mobility, the availability and use of appropriate manual-handling equipment, and a person to assist in the transfer (RCN 1996; NBPA 1998).

More recently, the UK National Minimum Standards for Care Homes for Older People (NMCS) (Secretary of State for Health 2001) require Care Home managers to ensure compliance with the Manual Handling Operations Regulations (1992) (MHOR).

Manual Handling Operations Regulations 1992

Under the regulations, employers are required to:
- avoid the need for employees to undertake manual handling operations which involve a risk of their being injured at work;
- make assessment of manual handling operations;
- take appropriate steps to reduce risk of injury to the lowest level which is reasonably practicable;
- give information to employees on manual handling operations.

Employees are required to:
- make full and proper use of any system provided.

Resident mobility

Policies that specify minimal lifting or no lifting in Care Homes can mean that residents become less mobile and increasingly dependent on mechanical hoists and devices. It is essential to balance such minimal or 'no-lift' policies with appropriate programs for rehabilitation, exercise, and walking.

'Minimal or 'no-lift' policies must be balanced with appropriate programs for rehabilitation, exercise, and walking.'

Maintaining the mobility of older people enhances their physical and psychological well-being and reduces the incidence of falls (Hauer et al. 2001). Maintaining a person's mobility also benefits the staff because residents become more independent and can assist nursing staff with tasks.

Mobility assessments and classification

There is a wide range of mobility and manual-handling assessment tools available from government authorities and as part of training systems and manuals. Care homes should have an agreed protocol for assessment of mobility and manual handling, and this should include the following features:

▶ clear, easy-to-follow steps or guidelines;
▶ clear linkage between a person's mobility chart and the manual-handling goals for that person;
▶ a section in which special behavioural requirements and precautions are noted; and
▶ accessible instructions and definitions on any 'subjective' components of assessments.

The protocol for manual-handling assessment should include a system for admission of people on weekends and evenings, so that interim manual-handling procedures can be put into place before a full assessment is available.

Some Care Homes also choose to have a 'quick-check' system available in the person's room. This might be a colour code or a single page of notes inside the wardrobe door. Confidentiality should not be compromised. Such a system assists temporary staff members in identifying the optimal manual-handling procedure for each person. However, such systems rely on information being current, on staff members being aware of the codes and symbols used in the notes, and on staff having the skills required to carry out the prescribed techniques.

Staff safety

It is important to assess the safety of all nursing tasks within any mobility program. For example, the mobility goal for a resident might be 'to maintain assisted walking', with the functional aim being 'assisted walking to the toilet'. However, if the person becomes unstable or unsafe, the risk of the nurse being injured increases. The task must then be modified, and a safe manual-handling procedure for toileting must be implemented (for example, a standing hoist). However, the mobility program should continue with modifications—for example, two carers can assist in sustained standing and exercises, with the aim of rehabilitating the person to his or her previous mobility status.

Minimising manual-handling injuries

Relevant strategies for minimising work-related musculoskeletal injuries from manual handling include:

▶ application of a risk-management approach (NBPA 1998; Worksafe Australia 1994) with demonstrable knowledge of procedures by workers and volunteers (MHOR 1992) (NMCS 2001);

▶ application and availability of appropriate mechanical lifting equipment and aids to eliminate manual lifting of people (Worksafe Australia 1994; RCN 1996; NBPA 1998; Varcin-Coad & Barrett 1998; Yassi et al. 2001);

▶ appropriate knowledge and manual-handling skills (NBPA 1998; Varcin-Coad 1999) including training in appropriate postures and movement patterns for the tasks (Burgess-Limerick 2003);

▶ minimal or no-lift policies and protocols for people-handling tasks, except in emergency or exceptional circumstances (RCN 1996; NBPA 1998); and

▶ encouraging the older person to assist in transfers as much as possible (NBPA 1998) regardless of real or perceived time pressure.

With regard to the last point, it should be noted that staff members are, in general, increasingly under pressure to perform tasks in a context of increasing resident dependency.

Manual-handling training
Principles

If nurses know when and how to apply appropriate equipment, techniques, and other risk controls, staff injuries can be decreased significantly (Varcin-Coad & Stewart 1999; Yassi et al. 2001). However, given the cost and time involved in skills training, the content of such programs should be appropriate to the facility and relevant to staff and residents.

Manual-handling training should:

▶ be delivered flexibly;

▶ employ effective techniques for adult learning;

▶ be in accordance with legislated requirements and competencies;

▶ be in accordance with the principles of risk management; and

▶ address issues of sustained postures and repetitious bending between waist and knee height.

The 'freestyle technique' is a non-prescriptive approach to safe manual handling (Varcin-Coad 1999, 2003). This technique develops the carer's internal body awareness and encourages the perception of a personal 'ideal' body position in terms of load and force in a variety of tasks. This concept, based on a risk-management approach, encourages every transfer or lift to become a potential learning experience, rather than a prescribed technique.

Content

Training should cover the importance of an ergonomic approach and the importance of back care and posture:

- ◗ current legislation and professional guidelines;
- ◗ risk assessment;
- ◗ dealing with unpredictable occurrences;
- ◗ local policies;
- ◗ handling strategies for clients with impaired mobility;
- ◗ safe management of inanimate loads;
- ◗ equipment use (including contraindications and safety issues); and
- ◗ problem solving.

(**National Back Exchange 2001**)

New staff

All new staff members require orientation before commencing hands-on work. Before working independently, it is best if they can have an opportunity to observe others, and then work on supervised shifts.

Orientation of new staff with respect to manual handling should include awareness of:

- ◗ the organisational policies, protocols, and systems that are in place;
- ◗ risk-management procedures;
- ◗ application of safe and effective manual-handling techniques related to the work area;
- ◗ related legal requirements; and
- ◗ organisational statistics, goals, and so on.

Existing staff

Training for existing staff and volunteers varies—depending on such factors as availability of time, competence of staff, and trends in incidents and injuries. Minimum training should include revision and assessment of knowledge of:

- ◗ risk-management systems and protocols, including care plan and assessment systems;
- ◗ how to seek assistance, report problems, manage equipment faults, administer first aid, report hazards and incidents, and so on;
- ◗ safe and effective use of relevant manual-handling equipment; and
- ◗ safe and effective manual-handling techniques related to the work area.

Frequency of training

All staff members should receive training and assessment in manual-handling skills at least annually (although every three months is preferable). Extra training is required when new equipment is introduced, when staff members return from injury or absence, and if workplace records indicate specific problems. Staff from other service areas (for example, maintenance and security) should also be included in risk-management and manual-handling training programs.

In the UK, employers are required to provide training during working hours. Sufficient follow-up by management must ensure safe supervision and monitoring of handling practice. Manual handling co-ordinators or link workers who are competent practitioners could be used to support staff further in the workplace.

Manual-handling training

Manual handling training should take account of:

* principles;
* content (new staff; existing staff; frequency of training; advanced skills);
* the role of management;
* the role of the manual-handling coordinator; and
* equipment and manual-handling aids.

All of these topics are discussed in detail in this chapter.

Role of management

The successful implementation of programs in mobility and manual handling requires significant commitment from management. An infrastructure needs to be established, and time and people must be allocated to develop a process that is appropriate to the particular facility.

Management should:

❱ oversee the development and writing of relevant policies and procedures specific to the facility and its residents;
❱ direct the implementation of the policies and procedures;
❱ appoint a manual-handling coordinator;
❱ monitor and review the process that is implemented;
❱ facilitate liaison among: (i) manual-handling personnel; (ii) the occupational health and safety team; and (iii) residents;
❱ provide time and resources for staff training; and
❱ provide ongoing support.

Longer-term compliance and management support can be assisted by including performance indicators within the personnel review system. For example, supervisors might be required to have 100% of new staff members complete a documented orientation program, and 50% of existing staff members attend skill sessions per month.

Resourceful management can transform a dissatisfied injury-ridden staff group into a happy, proactive, effective team.

> 'Resourceful management can transform a dissatisfied injury-ridden staff group into a happy, proactive, effective team.'

Manual-handling coordinator

The manual-handling coordinator might come from a nursing background, or from a related therapeutic background (such as physiotherapy or occupational therapy). Regardless of the person's precise background, the coordinator should have specialist knowledge in the care of older people and be aware of the relevant legislation, risk management, training and assessment, and manual-handling techniques. The coordinator might be the sole trainer and assessor in a facility, or might be the supervisor of a team of internal facilitators.

The duties of the coordinator should include:
- organising the orientation system and documentation;
- organising ongoing manual-handling and skill-training sessions;
- training and assessing documentation, collation, and review;
- problem-solving of manual-handling tasks and incidents;
- equipment monitoring, review, and trial;
- compliance audits;
- liaising with the health-and-safety team;
- reviewing manual-handling policy and procedures, and ensuring compliance with relevant legislation;
- communicating with all relevant staff members within the aged-care facility; and
- coordinating any workplace rehabilitation and return-to-work programs.

Equipment and manual-handling aids

There is a vast array of mechanical equipment available for Care Homes, and numerous manufacturers, models, attachments, and updates. However, minimum equipment requirements include hoists with a variety of slings, tilting shower chairs, and sliding sheets.

Problems of application and compliance can emerge with the introduction of any new equipment. Some of these problems can be avoided if staff members have been included in the trial and application of different models of equipment, and if their opinions have been taken into account and genuinely valued.

New equipment should be assessed against the criterion of whether it will make manual handling 'easier' and 'lighter' for staff. Equipment that is complicated or time-consuming should be carefully assessed against this criterion. All equipment should therefore be trialled in the clinical setting before purchase. These trials should involve at least two examples of the manufacturer's equipment. It is often necessary to trial two or three variations of the equipment, as well as performing a comparison between brands.

> 'New equipment must be assessed against the criterion of whether it will make manual handling 'easier' and 'lighter' for staff.'

Non-mechanical aids have also become more widely used in aged care to assist with mobility and manual handling. Research has indicated that sliding, pushing, or pulling a resident produces less spinal stress on the nurse than lifting (Garg et al. 1991). Therefore any product that promotes sliding, pushing, or pulling is likely to decrease the incidence of musculoskeletal injuries for staff and residents. In this regard, *slide sheets* (or 'slip-sheets') and *manual-handling walk belts* (or 'gait belts') are worthy of special mention.

Slide sheets

The introduction of slide sheets has successfully eliminated 'in-bed' lifts of residents in Care Homes.

Slide sheets are a type of sailcloth with a silicon (or similar) coating to decrease frictional forces associated with pushing, pulling, and turning tasks. However, due care needs to be taken to ensure that the hands and forearms of staff members are not placed at risk—as can occur if too much drag is applied during the sliding technique (Varcin-Coad 2003).

Every resident and situation brings variations to care plans, equipment, and techniques. Table 10.1 (page 131) is a 'quick-check' problem-solver for some of the more common problems associated with slide sheet use in Care Homes.

Table 10.1 Common problems associated with slide sheet use

Problem	Check
Staff say slide sheet does not work	if slide sheet is sufficiently slippery and the correct size; if two slide sheets are being used, or slide sheet on slippery surface; (two slide sheets should be used lengthwise for people: > 75 kg; resistive; high tone; cannot bend knees; no head control); if still lifting with slide sheet instead of sliding; (this can be a habit from draw or sling lifts); if staff members have sufficient skill in the use of slide sheets to problem-solve with a variety of residents and mattresses within facility.
Staff getting overuse injuries or pain in wrist or forearm	if slide sheet is sufficiently slippery; (commercial washing reduces slipperiness and continual purchase of new products is required); if still lifting with slide sheet instead of sliding; if the top sheet is being used to move person; (one layer slides over the bottom layer); if hand grasps thick (e.g., rolled-up foam or cloth within slide sheet) and close to person; if slide sheet pre-tensioned before slide; if person can assist during transfer; if sufficient slide sheet under dependent body parts of person
Staff say slide sheet pulls out when trying to turn person	if slide sheet is sufficiently slippery and correct size; if the top of the slide sheet is pulled at a 45-degree angle (rather than upward or parallel to surface); if the person tried to assist by lifting up at the time of the roll; (person should stay in contact with the sliding surfaces so the slide occurs between the slide sheets); if the second nurse is assisting the roll with gentle pelvic pressure and limb support during roll; (slide sheet must be tucked away from shoulder and elbow).
Staff not using slide sheets	if the slide sheets are readily available and accessible for staff; (minimum one per dependent person in bed, plus extras for washing); if there has been sufficient small group skill training and problem-solving sessions; (skill training should address appropriate skills for people within the unit);

(Continued)

Table 10.1 Common problems associated with slide sheet use *(Continued)*

Problem	Check
Staff not using slide sheets	if there is sufficient staff (and trainer) knowledge on the directions of movement that optimise transfers with slide sheets; (slide sheets should be no lift); if there is sufficient staff involvement with implementation and whether management is encouraging safer work practices (a protocol might be needed making slide sheets a mandatory requirement).
Resident will not use slide sheet	if consent was obtained initially; if person was given the opportunity to assist in the transfer; if the technique made it painful for the resident (e.g. too fast; lift instead of slide can cause skin discomfort; incorrect removal; poor technique to put slide sheet in); if there was appropriate communication with the person on initial application; if re-approach is necessary with more senior staff.

Author's creation (Varcin-Coad 2003)

Manual-handling belts

Manual-handling belts (walk belts or gait belts) aim to decrease the stress and strain associated with assisted standing techniques. In some cases they have been prescribed to eliminate 'hook-through' arm holds and to minimise skin trauma to residents (NBPA 1998). Sometimes they are called 'lifting belts'. However, this term should be avoided in facilities that are promoting a 'no-lift' policy.

Walk belts are usually 10–20 centimetres wide and have 2–4 vertical handles. The fastener is either a buckle or made of Velcro. A variety of brands or types is usually required to meet staff preferences and variations in residents' needs. Different training systems utilise variations in techniques with respect to use, direction of movement, and handholds.

'It is important that a skilled therapist assesses movements of staff during 'sit-to-stand' transfers.'

Whichever technique nurses use, due care needs to be taken to ensure that lifting, dragging, or pulling does not occur on the belt—except in emergency situations (for example, in controlling falls).

It is important that a skilled therapist assesses movements of staff during 'sit-to-stand' transfers. This assessment will ensure that staff members are not:

▶ lifting or dragging (instead of guiding or pushing);
▶ taking undue strain through their backs or upper bodies;
▶ twisting with the movement;
▶ performing a lifting action with their arms (thereby taking excess load on their shoulders and rotator cuffs);
▶ over-gripping with hands;
▶ placing residents' skin integrity at risk;
▶ transferring without allowing the person to assist;
▶ transferring without communicating with the resident or colleague; or
▶ transferring without due concern to the person's privacy and dignity.

Table 10.2 (below) is a 'quick-check' problem-solver for some of the more common problems associated with the use of walking belts in Care Homes.

Table 10.2 Common problems associated with walk belt use

Problem	Check
Belt slides up	if only one hand being used on belt (unless controlling a fall to the floor); if the belt is the correct size; if the belt is attached correctly; if the belt is being used as a lifting aid instead of a transfer aid; if the person is being transferred upwards rather than in an oblique direction.
Staff not using the belt	if the belt is available and accessible for staff; if there are sufficient small group training and problem-solving sessions (e.g. how to use a belt without lifting); if there is sufficient staff (and trainer) knowledge on the directions of movement that optimise transfers with belts; if there are sufficient staff members involved in implementation of new manual-handling procedures (and whether a protocol is needed).
Staff hooking onto or under person's arm (even with the belt on)	if technique used for hand holds is not secure enough for staff; if there is negative staff attitude to new equipment and procedures; if resident weight-bearing is sufficient for task; if pulling or dragging on resident arm is habitual; (intense skills training and self-validation that new technique is 'lighter' might be required).

(Continued)

Table 10.2 Common problems associated with walk belt use (*Continued*)

Problem	Check
Resident refusal to wear the belt	if contraindications and precautions observed (non-weightbearing residents, fractured ribs, open wounds, drains and tubes; precautions should be undertaken with osteoporosis, hernia, PEG feeds, resistive behaviours); if participation and consent gained; if inappropriate communication with the person occurred on initial application; if staff members have used belt in lifting or awkward manner that has hurt resident; (senior staff might need to renegotiate a trial of various belts); if it has been emphasised that the belt is to make the transfer more comfortable and safe; (make use of any behavioural traits known to enhance compliance and teamwork with resident).

Author's creation (Varcin-Coad 2003)

Conclusion

Effective skills in mobility and manual handling are pivotal to the provision of quality nursing care for older people. Open and uninhibited communication among staff, health-and-safety representatives, and management optimises safe and effective risk-management and manual-handling practices.

Nurses are constantly required to balance the needs (and requests) of residents with respect to mobility with the health and safety of staff. However, it is important to recognise that a happy, healthy nursing staff is essential to the overall health and happiness of those in their care.

Maintaining health-and-safety standards (such as avoiding the manual lifting of residents) is attainable, and this should be a primary goal for caregivers for older people.

Chapter 11

Wandering

Elizabeth Beattie

Introduction

Nurses who work with older people are familiar with individuals in residential care who are described as 'wanderers'. Episodes of wandering that result in a person being lost or injured are a common cause of admission to residential care, and caregivers around the world have identified wandering as a significant cause of stress to staff and families (Rockwood, Stolee & Brahim 1991).

Typical 'wanderers' are people who:

▶ become lost in familiar places;
▶ wait by the door wanting to leave;
▶ follow staff members, visitors, and other residents;
▶ enter other residents' rooms uninvited; and
▶ have difficulty resting.

The most obvious characteristics of these people are:

▶ higher activity levels than those of other residents;
▶ lack of conscious control over activity and rest; and
▶ resistance to distraction from their urge to be physically active.

The challenge for nurses and other caregivers is to respond, in a humane and dignifying manner, to the needs of people with high physical activity levels and spatial disorientation.

Unfortunately, a stigma is attached to wandering behaviour, and people can be labelled as 'difficult' or 'problematic'. These negative words suggest that the person is responsible for behaviour—such as becoming lost, resisting personal-care procedures, or elopement—over which they actually have little or no control. Because many people who wander have significant memory loss related to dementia, the view that people who wander are being difficult or problematic is both wrong and misleading—implying that the resident is able to stop the behaviour at will. Nurses who understand that people who wander have little or no control over their behaviour are in a better position to provide enlightened care.

> 'A stigma is attached to wandering behaviour, and people can be labelled as "difficult" or "problematic".'

Research about wandering has provided much useful knowledge about the phenomenon—including describing and measuring wandering, and identifying factors that contribute to wandering and wandering outcomes. Studies have challenged the notion that wandering should be managed by restriction and control (Algase et al. 1997), and many studies have identified the detrimental effects of physical and chemical restraint (Siegler et al. 1997). Indeed there are many positive effects of physical exercise for residents who wander.

Defining wandering

Due to the complexity of the behaviour, clinicians and researchers have had difficulty in defining 'wandering'. Despite the complexity of the behaviour, adopting a universal definition does help to promote conceptual understanding. The definition of wandering proposed by the present author and colleagues, and accepted by the North American Nursing Diagnosis Association, is as follows (NANDA 2002):

> . . . locomotion (with dementia or brain injury) characterized by its frequency and persistence; course appears to be meandering, aimless, or repetitive; frequently incongruent with boundaries, limits, or obstacles; impaired navigational ability.

Persons who wander

As many as a third of ambulatory nursing-home residents with a medical diagnosis of dementia might wander (Algase 1999a, 1999b), but accurate statistics are unavailable. Despite the absence of accurate data, there are some simple guidelines to follow when assessing an individual resident's tendency to wander. Nurses should be aware that any person whose main reason for being in residential care is a memory problem that prevents the person from living independently might have a tendency to wander.

'Any person with a memory problem that prevents the person from living independently might have a tendency to wander.'

Residents who might wander should be identified before admission, or at the time of admission. A tendency to wander can be indicated by:

- a history of wandering before admission to residential care;
- a medical diagnosis of any type of dementia (particularly Alzheimer's disease or multi-infarct dementia);
- a pattern of using physical activity to cope with stress;
- a social and outgoing personality before illness;
- recent relocation from another room, facility, or home; and
- robust physical health.

A model of wandering

A need-driven behaviour model has been designed by nurses to explain factors that might influence the development and occurrence of wandering and other behavioural disturbances (for example, aggression and disruptive vocalisations such as screaming) associated with dementia (Algase et al. 1996). The model (see Figure 11.1, below) suggests that there are relatively stable personal

Figure 11.1 Factors affecting need-driven behaviours

Background factors	Proximal factors	Need-driven behaviour
Neurological	Personal	Wandering
Cognitive	Physical environment	Physical aggression
General health	Social environment	Vocalisations

Adapted from Algase et al. (1996)

characteristics (background factors) that interact with more dynamic environmental factors (proximal factors) in individuals with dementia to produce behavioural disturbances. According to this model, wandering might be generated from an immediate resident need and be expressed in a way that is affected by the resident's stage of dementia and the environment.

The importance of a wandering history

It is important to undertake a systematic assessment of factors that might influence wandering behaviour in individual people. Many people have significant memory and language problems that make it difficult to communicate their needs. If a history of wandering can be established from a reliable informant, this should be explored in detail (Costa & McCrae 1988).

When discussing earlier wandering, nurses should ask about wandering behaviour in the context of where the person was living before coming into care. Nurses should enquire about wandering in familiar surroundings (within and around the home), as well as wandering in unfamiliar places. They should ask about whether the person left without supervision, whether he or she became lost, the duration of absences, and the mode of return. Answers to such questions provide an indication of the frequency, duration, and risk level of earlier wandering.

Wandering can be dangerous both in the home and outside. Wandering outside can obviously be dangerous because the person is exposed to the weather, busy roads, railway tracks, and so on. Inside the home, people who wander are exposed to electricity, stairs, and sharp objects—and the function of these potentially dangerous items might no longer be evident to them.

'Wandering can be dangerous both in the home and outside.'

Insights into a person's wandering history can help nurses to anticipate issues, and to solve problems. Examples of such insights might be a daughter commenting that her father never goes out without his hat, or a husband knowing that his wife loves to sit near water and trees. Informal caregivers are thus a rich source of potential management strategies.

Even if a history of wandering is not present, a person might develop wandering behaviour. Nurses need to be especially attentive if the person has one or more of the attributes previously mentioned (see 'Persons who wander', page 137). Any early evidence of wandering should be taken seriously, and not be dismissed as a 'one-off' incident. A single wandering episode can be fatal.

Assessing factors that influence wandering

General neurological status

There are two aspects of general neurological function that might influence wandering: (i) circadian rhythm; and (ii) motor functioning.

Circadian rhythm deteriorates with both normal ageing and dementia, and this deterioration can influence behaviour including wandering behaviour (Satlin et al. 1995; Algase et al. 1997).

Motor ability (which includes gait, balance, and motor strength) obviously affects behaviour and the performance of certain functional skills. Because motor ability remains intact late into the disease process in dementia, it is possible for residents to be walking independently but navigating inaccurately. The result is wandering behaviour. Eventually, a decline in motor ability reduces or stops wandering. However, in the interim, wanderers are at high risk of accidental falls, bruising, and fractures.

Assessment of neurological function

In assessing neurological function, nurses should:
- assess functional motor ability and walking safety using a gait-and-balance assessment tool;
- monitor those in their care to ensure that they are correctly using walking aids;
- assess all environmental safety hazards; and
- monitor medication—especially the dosage, timing, and side-effects of prescription sedatives and tranquillisers; any problems with excessive daytime drowsiness, night waking, or night wandering should be reported.

Cognitive impairment

People who wander have reduced cognitive performance—both globally and on many separate cognitive functions (such as memory, language, and visual–spatial tasks) (Algase 1999b; Burns, Jacoby & Levy 1990).

Cognitive impairment can be assessed using the mini-mental status examination (Folstein, Folstein & McHugh 1975) or the Mattis dementia rating scale (Mattis 1976). The global deterioration scale, a 7-point observational rating scale, is useful for determining the stage of dementia (Reisberg et al. 1988). The descriptions on the scale identify points in the progression of dementia from early stage to late stage.

The cognitive profile provided by these three tests can help nurses to understand the extent of cognitive limitations with which the resident is dealing, as well as the person's preserved abilities. However, these tests are only an indication of a person's status. Cognitive tests, taken alone, cannot determine the functional status of a person in any respect—including the functional development and expression of wandering behaviour.

Assessment of cognitive function

In assessing cognitive function, nurses should:
- take a baseline cognitive profile on admission;
- use a staging test to determine the stage of dementia;
- monitor the level of cognitive impairment and stage of dementia every three months, or after a major relocation; and
- focus on level of memory and attention function, visual–spatial skills, perseveration, and level of activity.

Personality

People who wander are likely to have experienced high stress levels (for example, marital separation, a life-threatening experience, financial problems, or immigration) during their lives, and are more likely to be people who used physical activity to cope with stress (Monsour & Robb 1982).

Assessment of personality

In assessing personality, nurses should:
- investigate the person's pre-illness personality and lifestyle preferences using informant interviews and the NEO 5-factor personality inventory; and
- identify previously enjoyed occupational, social, and leisure activities, and incorporate these into the person's routine.

General health status

Wandering can be affected by various health conditions (for example, infection), that leave a person feeling unwell. People with minor health problems are robust enough to continue wandering in the later stages of dementia, but such people are at higher risk of injury.

Anxiety and agitation have both been associated with wandering, and both can occur as part of dementia or of another general medical or psychiatric condition. The most commonly under-diagnosed psychiatric condition associated with dementia is depression, and depressed residents have a greater tendency to wander.

'Depressed residents have a greater tendency to wander.'

Assessment of general health status

In assessing general health status:

- assess general health status with a complete nursing history, including an assessment of co-morbid diseases;
- assess agitation using the Cohen-Mansfield agitation inventory (Cohen-Mansfield, Marx & Rosenthal 1989), or the agitated behaviour in dementia scale (Logsdon et al. 1999); and
- assess depression using the short geriatric depression scale (Sheik & Yesavage 1986).

Physical comfort

Physiological needs such as hunger, thirst, micturition, and defaecation are powerful behavioural motivators that operate independently of conscious control. People might wander seeking satisfaction of these needs. They might also wander as a result of pain, sleep disturbance, and other causes of discomfort.

Assessment of physical comfort

In assessing physical comfort:

- monitor verbal and non-verbal behaviour that might indicate an unmet need (for example, a person asking when meals are scheduled, asking for toileting, picking up empty cups and trying to drink, taking food off lockers, or grimacing or wincing in pain);
- record mealtime intake, snacking behaviour, pattern of toileting, pain medication profile, and so on;
- use a pain tool tailored to residents with dementia (such as the checklist of non-verbal pain indicators)(Feldt 2000);
- monitor sleep and daytime napping to identify a resident's pattern of sleep and rest over a one-week period; and
- examine the relationship between the verbal and behavioural expression of needs, and the occurrence of wandering episodes.

Physical and social environmental factors

Aspects of the physical environment can be modified to ameliorate wandering (Algase et al. 1997). Several aspects of the physical environment—including level of ambient light, the complexity of the design of the resident's living space, noise

'Aspects of the physical environment can be modified to ameliorate wandering.'

levels, and temperature—are being evaluated to determine the impact on wandering.

There is evidence to suggest that the staff mix in residential care, as well as the social milieu of the residence and the communication between residents and staff, can increase or inhibit wandering (Kolanowski 1995).

Observing wandering

Geographical pattern

One of the most useful ways to observe and describe wandering behaviour is to focus on patterns of behaviour. Four 'travel patterns' have been identified in ambulation among nursing-home residents with dementia (Martino-Salzman et al. 1991):

◗ direct (from point A to point B);
◗ pacing (backwards and forwards);
◗ lapping (in circuits); and
◗ random (no recognisable pattern).

Direct ambulation is not really 'wandering' behaviour. Even very impaired residents can display direct ambulation. Pacing is the least common pattern. It does not seem to be affected by the level of cognitive impairment; rather, it seems to be more related to anxiety or agitation. Lapping could represent a 'way-finding' strategy or a form of perseveration. The random pattern is the most disorganised pattern and occurs most often in more impaired residents.

Staff report

The Algase wandering scale (Algase et al. 2001) is a scale specifically designed to measure wandering in long-term care settings. The scale covers items specific to wandering: dimensions of persistent walking; spatial disorientation; eloping; shadowing; and routine walking. It provides caregivers with a complete profile of the resident's wandering behaviour from which to plan care.

Conclusion

As research into wandering develops, more insights about this complex phenomenon are being gained. The driving force behind these efforts is a desire to bring theory-driven, empirically tested interventions to nurse clinicians, so that they can better manage this vulnerable group of people in their care.

Chapter 12

Dysfunctional Behaviour

Graham A. Jackson and Colin MacDonald

Prevalence and definitions

Dysfunctional behaviour of various forms can present challenges to nurses who care for older people. In particular, so-called 'aggressive behaviour' can present difficulties, especially among elderly people who have cognitive impairments, such as those produced by dementia. Many studies have been carried out to establish the prevalence of aggression, but reported rates vary considerably—

from 18% to 65% (Ballard et al. 2000). One factor producing such a wide variation in incidence is that there is no consistent definition of what 'aggression' really is.

This problem of the definition of 'dysfunctional behaviour' in general, and 'aggressive behaviour' in particular, is not only important in terms of statistics. It is also important in

'A person who is labelled as 'dysfunctional' or 'aggressive' is less likely to receive respect and empathy, and is less likely to be listened to and helped.'

terms of how people are perceived, and how others respond to them. In any walk of life, if a person is labelled as 'aggressive', that label affects how others perceive and respond to that person. A person who is labelled as 'dysfunctional' or 'aggressive' is less likely to receive respect and empathy, and is less likely to be listened to and helped. If a person receives a label of 'aggressive', the provision of good-quality nursing care to that person can be seriously compromised.

The Oxford dictionary defines aggression as: '1. An unprovoked attack; an assault, 2. Behaviour intended to injure another person' (NSOED 1997). In the context of care of older people, one widely quoted definition is that aggressive behaviour is: 'an overt act, involving the delivery of noxious stimuli to (but not necessarily aimed at) another organism, object or self, which is clearly not accidental' (Patel & Hope 1992). These and similar definitions imply that an 'aggressive person' is intentionally hostile. However, in nursing older people, especially in the presence of dementia or other cognitive impairments, it can be difficult to be sure *exactly* what a person *really* intends. Both the persons involved and those caring for them can misinterpret intentions. The belief that dysfunctional behaviour is *intentional* can easily lead to mutual misunderstanding and intolerance.

Documentation and analysis

Whatever the precise definition, dysfunctional behaviour that could be described as 'aggressive' includes striking out, shouting in a threatening manner, swearing, throwing items around, biting, scratching, banging doors, and kicking. If this sort of behaviour is to be understood properly and managed professionally, proper documentation of such events is essential. This includes careful documentation of:
- a description of the behaviour;
- the situation in which it occured;
- the frequency and duration of such events;
- who was at risk (the 'aggressive' person, or others); and
- how the event was resolved.

Such careful documentation is essential if the behaviour is to be analysed and understood. In attempting such an analysis, nurses should ask themselves the following sorts of questions:
- What exactly is the problem behaviour?
- To whom is it a problem, and who is at risk?
- In what setting does it occur, and what are the precipitating factors?

▶ How often does it occur, how long does an event last, and how are such events resolved?

▶ How can the risk of such behaviour be minimised (for all concerned)?

Context and management

Most disruptive behaviours exhibited by elderly people with cognitive impairments are understandable in the context of the precise cognitive difficulties experienced by the people involved.

Disorientation in time and place commonly leads to a wish to leave—perhaps to go home, to go to an old address, or to leave for work. A nurse who tries to stop such activity by obstructing it might be perceived to be *in the way*. In these circumstances, it is no surprise that the person who is obstructed might shout, or try to push, or even hit out.

Disinhibition is a common feature of dementia—particularly if the frontal lobes of the brain are affected. This can lead to inappropriate behaviour—such as a reduced tolerance of others.

Agnosia (failure to recognise) can present particular difficulties. A person who believes that a Care Home is his or her previous family home might want others to leave—which can lead to disputes. An older person might also fail to recognise his or her spouse or child. If the way in which such relatives approach a resident is perceived by the person as being inappropriate, this can cause misunderstandings and distress.

Is there really a problem?

An older man in a nursing home had a minor misunderstanding with a visitor whom he did not recognise. A brief physical interaction followed. Although the incident was trivial, the visitor took serious offence and complained to nursing staff. The man's notes duly recorded that this man was a 'very aggressive' resident.

Unfortunately for this man, the visitor just happened to be a relative of a local general practitioner. Because the relative was inclined to take particular offence at the incident, the resident became permanently 'labelled'.

It is possible for a person to be labelled as 'very aggressive' as a result of an isolated incident of limited significance. The frequency and other relevant details of 'aggressive' behaviours should be carefully documented to establish that there really is a 'problem'.

Two perspectives on one incident

A man finds himself being taken to a strange unrecognisable place by a young woman who then tries to take off his trousers. He resists and a dispute threatens to erupt.

For the man, who suffers from agnosia, this is an unusual and frightening experience. He does not know this person, he does not recognise this place, and he cannot remember this having happened to him before.

For the nurse who is trying to take the man to the toilet, this behaviour has happened before. Indeed, it is typical of this difficult man who is 'known' to be 'aggressive'.

Labels of 'aggressive' can easily be applied to people who are thought to be difficult. Conversely, the label of 'aggression' is less likely to be applied to someone who has otherwise generally likeable traits.

Getting to know the person

It is important that nurses make an attempt to understand people who are supposed to be 'aggressive'. Nurses should gather as much information as possible about the person. They should enrol the assistance of family and friends who know the person better than anyone. Information should be gathered about the following aspects of the person in their care.

▶ *Previous personality*—some people might have been 'grumpy' or 'short tempered' all their lives. This has not changed due to ageing or illness, and is unlikely to be significantly changed by nurses now.

▶ *Previous lifestyle*—for a man who enjoyed football or rugby matches, shouting and swearing might have been accepted behaviour.

▶ *Previous social role*—someone who has always been in a dominant social role—as a father, a manager, a teacher (or even a nurse!) —might continue to exhibit this behaviour, and this can be interpreted by others as challenging, threatening, or even aggressive.

▶ *Life experiences*—successes, failures, and traumas can be significant, especially if these experiences include physical assault, abuse, imprisonment, or even rape. It is not difficult to understand why the approaches of nurses might be misinterpreted by someone who has had such experiences, and why an aggressive response might result.

▶ *Previous vocations*—in some jobs, aggressive behaviour might have been tolerated or even encouraged (for example, in the armed forces or manual labour).

What is 'normal'?

My father had an army background—which he never talked about. If startled while sleeping, or woken up too quickly, he would punch out! And yet my father was not an aggressive man! We had learnt to avoid this.

But we often wondered what would have happened if he had been admitted to hospital or a nursing home?

Identifying underlying reasons

Certain factors can make aggressive behaviour more likely to occur. In seeking to identify causes of such behaviour, nurses should consider factors in their own attitudes and behaviour, as well as considering factors in the person in their care. The following should be considered:

- attitudes of nurses and carers;
- care practices and routines;
- environmental factors;
- physical causes (illnesses, symptoms);
- other factors.

Each of these is considered below.

Attitudes of nurses and carers

Negative attitudes of nurses and carers can lead to poor tolerance of aggression. Nurses can have negative attitudes towards their work in general. They might view their work as being difficult, unstimulating, and unrewarding. This, in turn, can make it more likely that they will have negative attitudes towards those in their care.

Nurses might have ageist attitudes in which older people are viewed as dependent, a burden, and worthless to society. Some nurses might perceive older

Are you offended?

A nurse who had previously worked in a home for retired clergy was most offended when she began work in a new accommodation setting and came across a resident who tended to use swear words readily. Another nurse, who had previously worked in a nursing home in a working-class area with many ex-miners among the residents, did not think that the 'swear words' were at all unusual or offensive.

The attitudes, tolerance, and training of nurses all play a part in labelling a person as 'aggressive', and also play a part in how such behaviour is managed.

people in terms of certain stereotypes. They might, for example, feel that older

> 'If nurses have particular expectations and stereotypes of older people, those who fail to conform to these expectations can be viewed negatively.'

people should not swear, talk about sex, or behave aggressively (while tolerating such behaviour in younger people). Such attitudes and stereotypes can lead nurses to have a low tolerance of aggression. They can feel that people should not be allowed to get away with certain behaviour, and feel that something should be done. However, in society in general, standing up for oneself, protecting others, and even being aggressive (for example, in some sports) are often perceived as positive traits.

If nurses do have particular expectations and stereotypes of older people, those who fail to conform to these expectations and views can be viewed negatively. In turn, these people can react in an obstructive manner. When they do, they are labelled as being 'aggressive'.

Care practices and routines

Many aggressive incidents occur during direct personal care. Some nurses adopt a 'custodial approach' in which staff always 'know best'. In this approach, the emphasis is on power and control. Nurses have been overheard to say: 'When I'm on, he goes to his bed one way or another'. In such a culture, care is more likely to be based on punishment, isolation, or restraint. Rather than controlling aggressive behaviours, this approach only increases its severity and prevalence.

Routines in an organisation can lead to nurses adopting an inflexible approach in which all residents are perceived as having the same needs in terms of physical care. These goals of care are pursued irrespective of the views, feelings, and rights of particular individuals. Inflexible routines and the smooth running of the organisation become paramount—for example, with everyone having to be washed and dressed for breakfast at a particular time. If staff resources are limited, this increases the stress on nurses and reduces their tolerance of any behaviour that obstructs the completion of tasks on time. But such routines expect an individual person with dementia to change a lifetime's routines and way of life.

Environmental factors

For an older person with cognitive impairment, the internal environment of residential accommodation can be perceived in various ways. It might

---

An early riser

A man who had been a postman all his life was used to getting up between 4 am and 5 am. When he did this in hospital, the night staff felt that this was too early because he might wake other patients.

Nurses were adamant that this man was to go back to bed. A struggle followed, and one of the night staff was punched.

This man's life and care now changed. He was labelled as 'aggressive', and nursing attitudes to him were never the same.

---

be perceived as a hotel or as a prison. How the person behaves depends on this perception.

Too much noise can be disconcerting. This might come from televisions and radios, from people shouting (including carers), from domestic appliances, or from the clatter of pots and pans.

There might be too much stimulation. Carers, residents, and visitors can 'mill around' and confuse residents with too much activity and conversation. In many cases, such people are no more than 'strangers' to a person with dementia. Other residents can invade personal space. They can shout and make a noise, thus provoking 'dysfunctional' responses in others.

People can feel confined. Bedroom doors that are locked, 'no-go areas', and corridors that are shut off can effectively 'pen' people together—thus increasing the risk of conflict. There can be limited access to the outside—thus increasing a sense of frustration.

Physical illnesses and symptoms

Symptoms of illness can be unpleasant and distressing, and can increase confusion. An older person might not be able to communicate his or her symptoms verbally. Rather, such communication might be expressed through the person's behaviour and through his or her reactions to care routines. This might well be interpreted as 'dysfunctional' behaviour. For example, a person with painful knees might be unable to communicate his or her distress, but might resist if expected to walk down a corridor or to some other destination. Conversely, a person who is constipated or desperate to get to the toilet might pace about trying to find the toilet. But this person might be told by carers to sit down quietly.

Increased confusion might be caused by infection, anaemia, low blood glucose, or drugs. Such confusion might lead to 'dysfunctional' behaviour. Psychiatric disorders can produce hallucinations, delusions, or paranoid ideas.

Visual or hearing impairment can cause people to misinterpret conversations, background noises, or other people's actions.

Physical restraint can create anger, frustration, and resentment that becomes directed towards staff. This can increase the level and severity of aggression, which can become worse than the initial behaviour that led to the imposition of restraint.

Failing abilities can produce embarrassment, fear, and anxiety. People might become concerned about being forgetful or incontinent, or become anxious about being in an unfamiliar place surrounded by apparent strangers.

Faced with debilitating symptoms that they cannot understand or communicate, people can use 'aggression' as a form of communication or a defence mechanism. A person hitting out might effectively be saying: 'Leave me alone'.

Other factors

Other 'triggers' could be any act, stimulus, or environmental condition that causes or contributes to aggressive behaviour. By noting common patterns, themes, and circumstances, nurses can identify such triggers. Ways of removing or preventing triggers can then be considered to reduce episodes of aggression.

By considering antecedents, behaviour, and consequences ('ABC') possible triggers can be identified. The Box below illustrates such an 'ABC' tool.

ABC of identifying 'triggers'

The 'ABC' of identifying 'triggers' refers to *antecedents*, *behaviour*, and *consequences*. Nurses should ask themselves:

Antecedents

What was happening before the behaviour?

- Who was present?
- What was happening?
- Where did it happen?

Behaviour

What exactly happened?

- What was the person doing?
- Was it of sudden or gradual onset?
- Who or what was it directed at?
- How long did it last?

(Continued)

(Continued)

Consequences

What was the effect of the behaviour on the person or on others?

- What interventions were tried?
- What worked and what failed?
- Did the person calm down in his or her own time?
- Did the person cease the behaviour only after gaining something (food, drink, attention, or other comforts) ?
- Was any medication (sedation) or physical restraint used?
- Was anyone hurt or distressed by the behaviour?

Non-drug management
General principles

All nurses should be educated in the general principles of the non-drug management of dysfunctional behaviour, and should be equipped with specific strategies to use in particular situations (see also 'Staff education', page 156).

The general principles of management include the following:

- checking the history;
- following care plans;
- avoiding risk;
- knowing how to face aggression; and
- avoiding physical intervention.

The Box below provides information on each of these general principles of management.

General principles of managing dysfunctional behaviour

Checking the history

As noted earlier in this chapter, all incidents of dysfunctional behaviour should be carefully recorded, and nurses should check the history of aggressive incidents—severity, frequency, and circumstances. Who was involved? How many incidents have there been? How were previous incidents managed and resolved?

Following care plans

Nurses should follow any care plan instructions and guidelines. Nurses should be consistent, and should try not to deviate from approaches or strategies that are known to work with any given person.

(Continued)

(Continued)

Avoiding risk

Nurses should never put themselves in an 'at-risk' situation, especially if the person is known to be, or even potentially, aggressive. In particular, nurses should:

- not work alone (or, at the very least, should let someone know where they are);
- ensure that extra assistance is readily available, and someone can be contacted quickly if necessary;
- not work in confined areas; and
- be aware of possible triggers in their approach, and during personal care tasks with the person.

Facing aggression

If the person is becoming aggressive, nurses should stop and back off. They should ask themselves the following questions.

- Does this have to be done right now?
- Is there another way of doing this?
- Is it safe to leave the person?
- Are others safe—especially frail residents? (If not, these people should be removed from the vicinity.)
- Is assistance needed and, if so, how many people? (Too many can provoke an escalation of an aggressive reaction!)
- Is someone else better with this person (such as a carer or relative)?

Avoiding physical intervention

Nurses should never physically intervene or try to restrain a person unless absolutely necessary. To do this will only increase the risk of injury to the nurse and/or the person. Any good work already done in building a relationship of trust will be lost.

Many incidents of aggression occur in situations in which the person's body language and aggressive behaviour make it quite clear that he or she does not like what is happening and that there will be no cooperation. And yet carers often insist on continuing with the task, increasing the risk of injury to themselves or to the person.

Despite all efforts to avoid physical intervention, nurses might have to intervene physically and quickly in some 'flashpoint' situations to maintain the safety of the person and/or others. This should be limited to immediate safety needs, and should avoid any ongoing physical intervention, restraint, or confrontation—unless absolutely necessary.

Specific strategies

In addition to the general principles outlined above, nurses need specific strategies to deal with practical day-to-day situations.

When working with a person who is known to be aggressive, or is potentially aggressive, the main aim is to avoid provoking the person into an aggressive response. The aim is to help instil feelings of trust, confidence, and respect that will help to promote a better long-term relationship with the person.

Nurses should:

▶ approach from the front, use the person's preferred mode of address, introduce themselves, and adopt a non-threatening posture;

▶ use eye contact, be calm and unhurried in manner, speak in a clear and gentle voice, and use touch to reassure the person;

▶ use empathy and explain what they are going to do for the person rather than to the person;

▶ keep any instructions simple; assist and support the person to participate;

▶ respect the person's right to refuse and, if necessary, let another nurse try; and

▶ be consistent.

The Box below provides more information on these sorts of specific strategies

---

Specific strategies for managing dysfunctional behaviour

Nurses need specific strategies to deal with practical day-to-day situations. The main aim is to avoid provoking the person into an aggressive response by instilling feelings of trust, confidence, and respect. The following strategies will help in this.

- *Approach from the front*—nurses should *never* approach from the back or from the side of a person (because this can frighten or startle the person who might react by hitting out).

- *Use the person's preferred mode of address*—terms such as 'Pop', 'Gran', 'Sweetie', and so on can be perceived as disrespectful or humiliating.

- *Nurses should introduce themselves*—they should tell the person their names, and who they are (in their nursing role).

- *Adopt a non-threatening posture*—nurses should get down to the person's level, but should keep a safe distance (until they know the person well enough); towering over someone can be intimidating.

- *Use eye contact*—this is a powerful way of communicating trust; but 'staring someone out' can be interpreted as a threatening gesture.

- *Remain calm and unhurried in manner*—nurses should avoid sudden movements, and avoid showing any signs of tension or anxiety; people with cognitive impairments are often astute interpreters of non-verbal communication;

- *Speak in a clear and gentle voice*—nurses should avoid shouting, arguing, or any other form of confrontation.

- *Use touch to reassure the person*—but nurses should stop immediately if the person does not like this.

(Continued)

(Continued)

- *Use empathy*—nurses should imagine how they would feel if they were in this person's situation now.
- *Explain what they are going to do for the person rather than to the person.*
- *Keep any instructions simple*—nurses should use short sentences, with one question at a time.
- *Assist and support the person to participate*—for example, with respect to personal care, nurses should use skills of guiding and coaxing (and perhaps even mild coercion), but should avoid any form of physical restraint, holding, or grabbing.
- *Respect the person's right to refuse*—nurses can always return later.
- *If necessary, let another nurse try*—sometimes one nurse's face just 'does not fit', or reminds the person of someone else.
- *Be consistent*—if an approach/strategy works, it should be documented, and nurses should ensure that everyone does it this way.

Drug management

General drug use

Many drugs have been used to manage behavioural problems. The most commonly used drug, until fairly recently, was thioridazine (Melleril) —now no longer in use as greater awareness of its side-effect profile has developed (particularly its anticholinergic side-effects). Other drugs have included haloperidol (Serenace), chlorpromazine (Largactil), trazodone (Desyrel, Trialodine) (and other antidepressants), risperidone (Risperdal), anticholinesterase drugs such as donepezil (Aricept), and an assortment of others.

In the UK, in March 2004, the Committee on Safety of Medicines stated that risperidone or olanzapine should not be used for the treatment of behavioural symptoms of dementia, due to increased risk of stroke in older patients with dementia who are treated with these drugs.

Emergency drug use

There are some emergency situations in which drugs are required for behavioural problems. Such emergency situations are those that involve a significant risk of violence to others, or a severe degree of distress to the person being treated. Other ways of managing the situation should already have been tried, and failed. Medication should be used as a last resort. *Emergency* treatment should be for emergencies—it should never be something that is used routinely.

Neuroleptic drugs such as haloperidol, risperidone, or chlorpromazine have often been administered in such situations. However, in the UK, risperidone may now only be used for managing acute psychotic conditions in older patients who also have dementia, on a short-term basis and under specialist supervision (CSM 2004). Traditional antipsychotics may still be used, but all have potentially serious adverse effects including sedation, confusion, falls and tardive dyskinesia. They should only be used in the short term for treatment of severe psychosis, severe emotional distress, or behaviour that is dangerous to the individual or others. Low doses should be used, and individual patients monitored (The Royal College of General Practitioners 2004).

Examples include:

▶ lorazepam 0.5–2.0 mg;
▶ haloperidol 0.25–5.0 mg.

Prophylactic drug use

If aggressive episodes occur frequently despite all attempts to avoid or modify such behaviour, prophylactic medication can be considered.

There is a lack of evidence regarding best practice in this regard, but cholinesterase inhibitors may be of some benefit in behavioural and psychiatric symptoms. Other antipsychotics such as quetiapine 25–150 mg, sulpiride 100–1200 mg and amisulpride 50–400 mg may be tried (RCGP 2004).

Such drugs are relatively slow to act, and have a cumulative effect. Any drug prescribed should be given time to act. It should be prescribed initially at low dose, and increased only if necessary. At least a few days should have elapsed before changes are made. Drug administration should follow the axiom: 'Start low and go slow'. Such drugs should be used for as short a time as possible, and the need for ongoing administration should be continually reviewed.

Consent to drug use

In managing aggressive behaviour, the question of consent to treatment is often ignored. Aggressive behaviour, although sometimes due to agitation or distress, usually does not harm the 'aggressor', although it is potentially harmful to others. There is therefore an ethical question as to whether it is right to administer medication to cognitively impaired people, or to use other interventions, simply because of the effect of their actions on others. This ethical question becomes more complex if it involves administering drugs (or using other interventions) with people who are unable to give informed consent.

Medical treatment for aggression also presents a problem because the behaviour is usually of sudden onset, and of short duration. This often means that medication is given in anticipation of the possibility of 'trouble'. People are therefore sedated because they *might* sometimes annoy or even assault other people. This might, at first sight, appear to be reasonable. But this is not done

> 'Football hooligans are not sedated in anticipation of the possibility that they *might* harm others. Is it right to do so in aged care?'

with other people in the community. For example, football hooligans are not sedated in anticipation of the possibility that they *might* harm others. Is it right to do so in care of older people?

In all cases, the question of consent must be considered. As in all emergencies in medical and nursing practice, the requirement for consent can be overriden by the needs of the emergency. However, the issue of consent *must* be considered in every case.

Staff education
The cornerstone of management

The cornerstone to successful management of dysfunctional behaviour in aged care is adequate education of nurses and the provision of sensible strategies and hints. Caring for people who can be aggressive is no easy task. Education and training can:

▶ help nurses to develop a better general understanding (and tolerance) of dysfunctional behaviour in older people; and

▶ develop particular skills and instil confidence in individual nurses that they can safely and effectively manage difficult situations.

Education and training can prevent problems arising in the first place and/or facilitate a prompt response to any potentially aggressive situation before it develops into something more serious.

General principles

Staff training should emphasise that the keys to success are *observation*, *de-escalation*, and *intervention*.

Observation

Nurses should be aware of *who* needs to be observed, *where*, and *why*. It is obviously impossible to observe every person for every minute of the day. In any event, every person's right to privacy must be respected. Nevertheless, it is prudent to take reasonable steps. For example, the continual presence of a carer in a sitting room can result in more timely responses to potentially aggressive situations and can prevent harm or distress to others (especially to frail or vulnerable residents). Arrangements will vary from establishment to establishment, but prudent observation is the key to prevention.

De-escalation

The term 'de-escalation' refers to skills or technique that help to distract the person's attention or defuse a difficult situation. This covers a range of techniques—including verbal distraction, touch, reassurance, empathy, listening, and removing any obvious triggers. Good knowledge of the person is obviously very helpful in this regard.

Intervention

Apart from interventions aimed at de-escalation, as previously noted nurses might have to intervene physically and quickly in some 'flashpoint' situations to maintain the safety of the person and/or others. This should be limited to immediate safety needs, and should avoid any ongoing physical intervention, restraint, or confrontation—unless absolutely necessary.

Specific hints and strategies

Apart from the general principles of staff education noted above (and discussed elsewhere in this chapter), the following specific hints and strategies might be useful.

Hints for personal interaction

In dealing with people at the interpersonal level, nurses should:
- never work alone, or in a situation where assistance cannot be summoned;
- never put themselves or others in an 'at risk' situation;
- never approach a person from behind;
- avoid sudden movements;
- avoid confrontations and arguments;
- avoid any form of physical restraint;
- try to find the reason for the aggressive behaviour, rather than trying to control it; and
- de-escalate aggression at an early stage.

Hints for general care

Apart from the above hints dealing with personal interactions, the following hints on general strategies might prove useful in the care of people who demonstrate aggressive behaviour.

- *Flexible routines*—these should take account of the previous lifestyles and present needs of individual persons in care.
- *Environmental approaches*—these should aim to produce a 'homely environment' (with personal possessions and age-appropriate furnishings), the provision of quiet private areas and a general reduction of noise (with particular attention to television and radio volume), attention to lighting (good natural lighting to maximise visual ability and variable lighting to suit mood), and open-plan areas (where the person can see and be seen).
- *Involvement of relatives*—making use of their knowledge of the person, and involving them in a caring role (if appropriate).
- *Physical activities*— to burn off physical energy constructively (walking, domestic chores, or gardening).
- *Relaxation*—to decrease agitation and enhance calmness (music, hand massage, or simple rest in a chair or bed).
- *Distraction*—to divert attention away from any causative factors (invitation to go for a walk or join staff in a cup of tea; encouragement to go to a quieter and more private place).
- *Person-centred and consistent approaches*—respecting individual needs and recognising that what works for one person might not work for another.
- *Favourite carers*—utilising the fact that many people are more comfortable with a particular, nurse, or relative.

Conclusion

Rather than labelling behaviour (or, indeed, a person) as 'dysfunctional', nurses must identify particular incidents—including their frequency and their consequences. The use of the term 'aggressive' can, in itself, lead to a change in attitude to that person. This, in turn, can lead to poorer quality of care.

Management of such difficulties usually falls to those carers who have most 'hands-on' care. In a hospital or in a Care Home these staff members are often the least well trained, and might be the least experienced. It is important that all staff members dealing with older people receive regular training of good quality, and that they are well supported by their managers.

There is no *right* way to deal with problem behaviour. Each person, each carer, and each situation is different. Nurses must persevere, and solutions have to be tailored to particular events. It is not always possible to get it right. Nurses should not see a lack of success as being failure. Nurses fail their patients only if they do not try. The key is to persevere with care that is genuinely person-centred.

Chapter 13

Pain Management

Robyn Dealtry

Introduction

In recent years, significant strides have been made in all areas of pain management—including new treatment techniques, improved pain medications, and a better understanding of pain transmission. However, residents in Care Homes still suffer unnecessary pain. The ethical obligation to manage pain and to relieve suffering should be at the core of the nurse's practice (AHCPR 1992).

> 'The ethical obligation to relieve suffering should be at the core of the nurse's practice.'

Definition of pain

The International Association for the Study of Pain defines pain as: 'an unpleasant sensory and emotional experience associated with actual or potential tissue damage or described in terms of such damage' (IASP 1979).

Pain is very subjective, and the individual experience of pain depends on a variety of factors. These include (Hawthorn & Redmond 1998):

▶ cultural influences;
▶ gender;
▶ age;
▶ disease;
▶ previous experiences;
▶ socialisation;
▶ relief;
▶ distraction;
▶ socioeconomic status; and
▶ religious beliefs.

These factors should be considered when nurses are assessing pain and attempting to understand an individual's perception of his or her pain. The sensation of pain depends on the central nervous system, and a person's perception of an event as being 'painful' depends on the function of higher brain centres. Ultimately, pain is what the person says it is!

> 'Ultimately, pain is what the person says it is.'

Types of pain

Acute and chronic pain

Pain can be acute or chronic. *Acute pain* is of sudden onset and lasts for a short period of time. It is 'fast pain', transmitted by small myelinated nerve fibres. Examples include surgical and traumatic pain. In contrast, *chronic pain* (or persistent pain) is 'slow pain', and is transmitted by larger unmyelinated nerve fibres. It lasts for a longer period of time (six weeks or more). Examples include arthritis and back pain. Chronic pain might begin as acute pain and later progress to a persistent state. It can affect every facet of a person's daily living and quality of life.

> 'Chronic pain can affect every facet of a person's daily living and quality of life.'

Somatic, visceral, and neuropathic pain

Somatic pain arises from noxious stimulation of structures such as skin, tendons, joints, ligaments, and muscles. It is localised and definite, and is often described as being 'sharp' or 'stinging'. An example is pain from burns.

Visceral pain arises from noxious stimulation of abdominal organs, peritoneum, and pleura. It can be described as 'colicky', 'cramping', or 'aching'. An example is pain caused by distension of the bowel. This type of pain can produce autonomic nervous system responses—including changes in blood pressure and pulse, and associated nausea and vomiting.

Neuropathic pain (also called 'neurogenic pain') results from damage to the peripheral or central nervous systems. This type of pain can be very unpleasant and difficult to treat. It is often resistant to opioid analgesic therapy. Neuropathic pain can be described as 'burning', 'dull', 'aching', and 'boring'. Examples include postherpetic neuralgia, phantom limb pain, and pain from diabetic peripheral neuropathy. Neuropathic pain can also involve episodes of shooting pain (technically called 'lancinating pain') and the experience of paraesthesia (various forms of 'tingling' and significant discomfort). Lancinating pain and paraesthesia can be associated with tumour invasion, spinal cord lesions, and multiple sclerosis. Entrapment of nerves is a common cause of neuropathic pain. The prevalence of neuropathic pain increases with age.

Other types of pain in older people include:

▶ *allodynia*—a painful response to normally non-painful stimuli (such as light, touch, and cold);

▶ *hyperalgesia*—an exaggerated or excessive response to painful stimuli; and

▶ *central pain*—damage in the central nervous system caused by lesions of various types (for example, phantom limb pain or stroke).

Age-related factors

Older people do not always complain about their pain. They often feel that pain is synonymous with ageing and that they should accept it. Although pain is not an inevitable result of ageing, older people are at greater risk of many disorders that can produce pain (for example, arthritic disorders, cardiovascular disease, osteoporosis, and cancer). In addition, painful surgical procedures are common among older people, including operations to correct orthopaedic problems (such as fractures and degenerative joint disease) and operations for various forms of cancer (Pasero, Reed & McCaffrey 1999).

> ### 'My other leg is also 101 years old!'
>
> Some people mistakenly assume that pain is an inevitable part of ageing. The illogical nature of this misconception is best illustrated by the story of a 101-year-old man who complained that his left leg hurt.
>
> The physician suggested that this was to be expected in a man of 101 years. On hearing this, the old man considered the logic of the explanation. He then asked the physician to explain why his right leg, which was also 101 years old, did not hurt at all!
>
> **Adapted from Pasero, Reed & McCaffery (1999)**

There are many misconceptions about pain experienced by older people. It should not be assumed that (Pasero, Reed & McCaffrey 1999):

- pain is a natural part of growing old;
- pain perception decreases with age;
- opioids can stop the elderly from breathing, and should therefore be avoided; or that
- older people do not experience pain while sleeping.

Many physiological changes occur as a person ages. These changes include (Macintyre & Ready 2001):

- changes in brain tissue;
- decreased cardiac output;
- decreased neural transmitters and endogenous opiates;
- reduced liver function;
- reduced renal function;
- altered protein binding;
- concurrent diseases;
- lack of motility of the gastrointestinal tract resulting in constipation;
- decreased muscle bulk causing a decline in mobility and an increased possibility of falls;
- cognitive impairment resulting in poor communication; and
- visual and hearing impairment.

Factors influencing treatment of pain in older people include (Hawthorn & Redmond 1998):

- polypharmacy and drug interaction;
- fear of addiction (usually with opiates);
- fear of loss of control;
- fear of needles;
- fear of drug side-effects (especially with opioid analgesics);

- fear of masking physical signs and symptoms;
- individual variability in response to pain medication;
- non-compliance with treatment;
- poor nursing assessment; and
- low priority given to pain assessment and management.

Pain assessment

Complexity of problem

Pain is a complex subjective phenomenon. Features such as intensity, time course, quality, impact, and personal meaning should all be assessed. The reporting and documentation of pain is a social transaction between nurses and the older people in their care, and successful assessment and control of pain depend on establishing a positive relationship among healthcare providers, older people, and their families.

Self-reporting is the most reliable pain indicator, but self-assessment in older people can be a problem because older people are often stoic about their pain. In addition, people who are unable to describe their suffering—as a result of dementia, confusion, or other difficulties—pose a challenge to caregivers in assessing pain. In older people, common illnesses can present in unusual ways—for example, 'silent' myocardial infarctions and 'painless' intra-abdominal emergencies (Clinch, Banerjee & Ostic 1984; MacDonald 1984). Visual and hearing impairments are also common obstacles in self-reporting, and in the completion of pain scales.

> 'Inappropriate attitudes and underestimating pain in elderly people can deny them appropriate pain relief and an optimal level of activity.'

Inappropriate attitudes and underestimating pain in older people are other common barriers to achieving accurate assessments by nurses and carers. Inappropriate attitudes can deny many older people appropriate pain relief and an optimal level of activity.

Assessment and measurement tools

There are many scales, flowcharts, and questionnaires available for pain assessment. These include:

- daily pain diaries;
- pain flowcharts;

- face and colour scales (useful in paediatrics, aged care, and for non-verbal people);
- numerical scales;
- pain charts (body drawing);
- visual analogue scales (VASs);
- verbal descriptor scales (VDSs); and
- verbal distress scales (VDSs).

Documentation

Documentation is essential for effective assessment and re-assessment of pain. In addition, accurate documentation is required for:

- administration of analgesics and the management of side-effects of analgesia;
- management of pain behaviours and attention to a person's quality of life (including sleep, appetite, and concentration); and
- psychosocial, spiritual, and cultural aspects of pain management.

Guidelines for effective pain management
Principles

The objectives of pain management are: (i) the minimisation of physical deconditioning; and (ii) the maximisation of function.

In striving to achieve these objectives, it is important that nurses *believe* an older person's report of pain, and use appropriate language in discussing that pain (for example, 'pain' might be an inappropriate word in some circumstances; 'sore', 'hurts', or 'aches' might be more appropriate).

It is also important to intervene promptly and provide adequate relief before pain becomes severe. Frequent regular analgesia (around the clock) might be more appropriate for persistent pain, rather than 'as needed' medication. Drug regimens should be kept as simple as possible to aid compliance and to avoid drug interactions.

> 'It is important to intervene promptly and provide adequate relief before pain becomes severe.'

An effective drug should be used for particular types of pain. The World Health Organization analgesic ladder can be used as a guide for administering medications (WHO 2003). Nurses should be knowledgeable about the pharmacokinetics and pharmodynamics of analgesics. They should assess and reassess pain at regular intervals, and manage undesirable side-effects effectively (such as nausea, vomiting, constipation, confusion, and hallucinations).

Pain-relief measures should be modified according to the person's response, and the general rule of 'start low and go slow' should be observed in titrating to individual needs.

People in Care Homes, or their families, should be encouraged to keep a daily diary—which can be useful in gathering and comparing data. In addition, while caring for people who have communication difficulties, nurses should observe pain

> 'Observation of pain should be considered as "the fifth vital sign".'

behaviours carefully (such as limping, grimacing, and withdrawing from activities). Observation of pain should be considered as 'the fifth vital sign'.

One scale used to assess pain in people with advanced Alzheimer's disease consists of eight items: (i) noisy breathing; (ii) absence of an appearance of contentment; (iii) looking sad; (iv) looking frightened; (v) frowning, (vi) absence of a relaxed body posture; (vii) looking tense; and (viii) fidgeting. These items are examined over five minutes (McCaffery and Pasero 1999).

Depression and anxiety should be managed separately with appropriate medications. Complementary therapies should be used when appropriate, and spiritual needs and requirements should be explored and managed appropriately.

Nurses should strive for an acceptable level of comfort when total pain relief is not possible.

Pharmacological pain management

Older people require lower doses of analgesics because of altered pharmacokinetics (how a person deals with drugs) and pharmacodynamics (how a person responds to drugs).

Routes of administration

Analgesic agents can be administered by different routes—depending on the absorption and elimination of the drug, and the desired time of effect of the drug. Occasionally a particular route is chosen to enable direct delivery of a high concentration of a drug to a particular site (for example, an epidural or intrathecal injection) (DHS 1998).

Routes of administration of analgesia are:

- *oral:* this route is preferred as first-line management, if possible;
- *sublingual;*

▶ *rectal:* this route is particularly useful when the oral method is not possible (for example, when nausea and vomiting are present);

▶ *transdermal;*

▶ *intravenous:* this route is preferred for short-term, postoperative acute pain;

▶ *intramuscular:* this route of administration is painful, and absorption can be erratic if the peripheral circulation is diminished;

▶ *subcutaneous:* this is minimally invasive, and is useful for both chronic and cancer pain management; the subcutaneous route is not particularly useful in acute postoperative pain management because of diminished peripheral circulation;

▶ *epidural (epidural space)* and *intrathecal (subarachnoid space):* these are utilised for advanced cancer pain management, when conventional treatments offer no pain relief or cause side effects (for example, if opioids become unacceptable).

Types of analgesics

Paracetamol

Paracetamol is an analgesic and antipyretic drug that is indicated for mild-to-moderate pain and fever (for example, benign headache, arthritis pain, bone pain in cancer, and 'flu-like symptoms). Paracetamol has little anti-inflammatory activity, and can be used when non-steroidal anti-inflammatory drugs (NSAIDs) are contraindicated (for example, peptic ulceration, asthma, and renal failure).

Paracetamol is a useful adjunct to opioid therapy. A maximum dose of 4 grams per day (up to 6 grams per day in palliative care) is recommended. Paracetamol is contraindicated in liver failure, and liver function tests are required in the presence of liver damage, high alcohol intake, or poor nutritional status.

Codeine

Codeine is a mild opioid and therefore has a central action. It is indicated in mild-to-moderate pain—either alone or in combination with paracetamol. A dose of 30 milligrams of codeine is approximately equal to a dose of 6 milligrams of morphine.

Codeine can also be used as an antidiarrhoeal agent or as a cough suppressant. Because it has a constipating effect, stool softeners, adequate hydration, and a high fibre diet should therefore be considered when codeine is administered to older people.

Tramadol

Tramadol is indicated for moderate-to-severe musculoskeletal pain and neuropathic pain states. It can be useful in mild-to-moderate cancer pain, and in acute pain if aspirin, paracetamol, and NSAIDs are contraindicated.

In older people (more than 75 years), the dose should not exceed 300 milligrams in a 24-hour period. A reduced dose is recommended for people with moderate to severe renal impairment.

Compared with other opioids, tramadol causes less respiratory depression, less sedation, less constipation, and less abuse, and is therefore a useful alternative in older people. However, nausea, vomiting, dizziness, and orthostatic hypotension are potential hazards in older people.

Tramadol is contraindicted in older people already taking tricyclic anti-depressants or epilepsy medications, or those experiencing alcohol and drug withdrawal, metabolic disorders, and head trauma (AMH 2002).

Non-steroidal anti-inflammatory drugs (NSAIDs)

NSAIDs provide analgesic, anti-inflammatory, and anti-pyretic effects. They are therefore useful in the treatment of pain and inflammation of arthritis, and for the management of postoperative pain. Co-administration with opioids might be indicated for severe pain.

The risk of gastric bleeding and renal toxicity associated with the use of NSAIDs is increased among older people. A much lower dose is indicated in people with renal impairment, and the drugs are contraindicated in renal failure. There are many important drug interactions between NSAIDs and other medications commonly prescribed for older people—such as diuretics, anticoagulants, hypoglycaemic agents, and anticonvulsants.

The rectal method of administration is useful when a person cannot swallow, or when a prolonged action is desired (for example, overnight). NSAIDs can also be applied topically, and are widely used in this way for musculoskeletal pain.

Opioid analgesics

Opioid analgesics are used for moderate-to-severe pain. Morphine can also be used for the relief of severe dyspnoea—for example, in cases of lung cancer and terminal chronic obstructive pulmonary disease (COPD).

Active toxic metabolites can accumulate in older people with renal impairment—especially with pethidine. Pethidine should therefore be avoided in older people.

'Pethidine should therefore be avoided in older people.'

Fentanyl, a synthetic opiate that possesses inactive metabolites, is the most suitable drug for older people, especially those with renal impairment.

Opioids can produce cognitive and neuropsychiatric dysfunction. Older people should therefore be given lower initial doses of opioids, and the dose should then be gradually titrated to the optimum level.

Constipation is a significant problem with opioids. This is exacerbated by infirmity, inadequate fluid intake, reduced physical activity, and other constipating drugs (for example, tricyclic antidepressants, major tranquillisers, and diuretics). High-fibre diets, adequate fluid intake, and faecal softeners are advised for older people.

Non-pharmacological and complementary management

Complementary therapies are designed to be used in conjunction with traditional medicine, and not as a substitute. Complementary therapies and non-pharmacological approaches include:

▶ art and music therapy;
▶ relaxation therapy;
▶ massage;
▶ aromatherapy;
▶ magnet therapy;
▶ reiki;
▶ therapeutic touch;
▶ reflexology;
▶ pet therapy;
▶ behaviour management;
▶ acupuncture;
▶ shiatsu and acupressure;
▶ Bach flower remedies;
▶ hypnosis;
▶ cryotherapy; and
▶ transcutaneous electrical nerve stimulation (TENS).

Increased anxiety levels increase the level of pain sensation in older people, and the above therapies can assist in relieving physical and mental tension, and promoting a sense of well-being. Nurses have always used touch and massage in their daily caregiving—massaging necks, feet, hands, and backs using a variety of essential oils. Massage promotes relaxation, and results in lowered anxiety levels.

Conclusion

Pain is most often poorly managed in those who are most defenceless against it—the young and the old. Although great advances have been made in pain management in recent years, there is still much to be done—especially in the area of pain research. However, older people's nurses can do much to assist those in their care. An awareness of the theory and practice of modern pain management in nursing can do much to relieve suffering and promote well-being.

> 'Pain is most often poorly managed in those who are most defenceless against it—the young and the elderly.'

As John Dryden (1631–1700) once remarked: 'For the happiness mankind can gain is not in pleasure, but in rest from pain' (Dryden 2001)

Chapter 14

Palliative Care

Rosalie Hudson

Introduction

What practical nursing skills are required in aged care and what principles should be applied to end-of-life care for older people? What is the goal of palliative care in a nursing home or hostel? When should it be commenced? What are the options?

Given the demographic changes that are occurring in Western societies, especially the ageing of the population and the increase in chronic illness, nurses are challenged to consider these sorts of questions, and to re-think their perceptions of palliative care.

The aim of this chapter is not to cover in detail all the issues of practical management and symptom control for dying older people. Rather, the aim is to present a broad understanding of palliative care and its application in care for older people. Practical examples are given, together with two narratives that amplify the discussion of whether dying older people need palliative care. The broader aim is to counter the common perception that being in a nursing home is a 'fate worse than death' and the extreme view that suicide or euthanasia is a preferred option.

The changing demographic scene

Chronic diseases are now replacing diseases that would have previously resulted in an early death (Lynn 2001). There is now a demographic shift from life-threatening short illness to serious progressive disease. This provides a new challenge for nurses, particularly because the last phase of life can lead to significant disability in the years preceding death. There is a likelihood that an increasing number of older people will require long-term residential care, rather than short-term hospice palliative care. In spite of the trend towards healthy ageing and extended life expectancy, the prognosis for many people remains uncertain right up to the end of their lives. Health services need to accommodate this trend towards 'slow-dying' from progressive illness. As treatment for cancer and heart disease improves, so the incidence of chronic diseases (including conditions such as dementia) increases. These changes indicate that a different approach to palliative care is required—an approach in which the transition from 'cure to care' is now more variable than precise.

Goals for end-of-life care

Cicely Saunders, founder of the hospice movement, famously said: 'How people die remains in the memories of those who live on' (Saunders & Baines 1989). Although this statement might have been more frequently applied to younger people dying of cancer, memories of death and dying apply no less to the families of older people. The statement also applies to nurses who are committed to reflection on their practice and who try to ensure that end-of-life care is of the highest quality in every situation. And it also applies to those who are concerned about episodes of care that have been less than adequate. So, how do we set goals for improved care?

> 'How people die remains in the memories of those who live on.'

Rather than *generalising* about whether dying people need palliative care, the best way to approach this question is through the *particular*.

- What does this particular person need at this particular time?
- What are this person's expectations of residential care at the end of life?
- What changes have occurred in the person's physical, psychological, emotional, social, or spiritual needs?
- If this particular person is approaching death, what particular needs are identified and what is appropriate care in the context of this person's unique life history and future hopes?

‣ Have the family's hopes and expectations changed?
‣ What can this particular person's family contribute to a discussion on palliative care in this particular situation?

Planning

One of the basic principles of palliative care is that it should not be restricted to the last days or hours of life. Soon after the admission of each person, nurses should ensure that the person and family are aware of the context in which palliative care is provided. This should be discussed in a relaxed, informal manner, rather than as an interrogation with the ticking boxes on an assessment sheet. Just as good palliative care arises from good planning, so the initial discussion needs to be planned. Whether or not a specific palliative-care assessment form is used, the discussion should be clearly documented. Figure 14.1 (below) shows a useful assessment form, and Figure 14.2 (page 175–6) provides a helpful checklist for nurses to consider.

© (Example only: Rosalie Hudson & Associates 2003)

Palliative Care Assessment

Name: _____

(or resident label)

1. Has the goal of care changed to focus on comfort measures and symptom control rather than rehabilitation or curative measures? If yes, what collaboration has occurred? (e.g., doctor, family, resident, other)?

   _____

2. Have the goals of palliative care been explained to resident and family (including appropriate care of the family, options for visiting, etc.)?

   _____

3. What are the most important issues of palliative care for the resident and family?

   _____

4. Are there any cultural or spiritual issues not covered in other assessment forms?

   _____

5. Is referral needed to consultant palliative-care nurse or palliative-care physician (or other member of a palliative-care team)? Please specify:

   _____

6. Is there a comprehensive drug regimen in place to cover all relevant symptoms? Please specify:

   _____

(Continued)

(Continued)

7. If narcotics have been prescribed, are there sufficient orders and supplies to cover after hours and weekends?

_____

8. Have options for complementary therapies been explored with resident/family? Please specify:

_____

9. Has the changed goal of care been formulated into the care plan?

_____

10. Has the doctor's after hours availability been confirmed and clearly documented? Give details:

_____

11. Are there any other referrals appropriate, e.g., use of volunteers, allied health staff, chaplain? Please specify:

_____

12. Have options for single/shared room been explored? (e.g., check resident/family concerns and preferences) Please specify:

_____

13. Would the family welcome any literature on palliative care, e.g., use of narcotics, issues of dehydration? Please specify any literature provided:

_____

14. Have the resident's end-of-life wishes/choices/options been discussed and recorded? Please specify:

_____

15. Are there any staff concerns about providing palliative care for this resident (e.g., further education/information/discussion required)? Comments:

_____

16. Are there any other issues the resident/family would like to discuss?

_____

17. Have options been explored for further review as circumstances change (e.g., family meeting)?

_____

Name of person completing this form (BLOCK LETTERS) _____

Date _____

Figure 14.1 Palliative-care assessment form

Rosalie Hudson & Associates (2003); published with permission

Palliative Care Nurse Checklist

(for use with Palliative Care Assessment Form)

Good palliative care relies on professional nurses' advance planning. This checklist is not exhaustive but might serve as a prompt. Palliative care relies on a team approach rather than one nurse making independent judgments (except of course in the case of emergency).

Advance planning

1. Before contacting the doctor, consult with colleagues and *write down* a list of requirements, to avoid unnecessary phone calls and to ensure consistency of communication.
2. Wherever possible, the doctor should be involved with the nurse, resident, and family in *planning* the palliative care in accordance with agreed goals.
3. Consult relevant drug guides and pharmacological information to ensure quality use of medicines and to ensure informed discussion with doctor, based on best practice.

Checklist for nurse–doctor communication

1. Obtain order for relevant medications *in advance*, including options when oral administration no longer appropriate.
2. Ensure sufficient orders for breakthrough pain.
3. Order *in advance* for appropriate medication to control secretions (if necessary).
4. Is treatment for anxiety required, or other drug(s) for terminal restlessness?
5. Is the resident prescribed any unnecessary drugs, which could be *ceased*?
6. If oxygen is considered, discuss with doctor *first*. Oxygen is not *necessarily* an effective adjunct to palliative care.
7. Are any other prescriptions required (e.g., for mouth care, skin care)? (*Beware of prescriptive mouth-care agents when cool water might suffice, but check for painful fungal infection, etc.*)
8. Explore options for continuous subcutaneous infusion if required.
9. If narcotics are prescribed, what adjuvant drugs are needed (e.g., anti-emetic, laxative)?
10. Discuss appropriate use of nasopharyngeal suction *and consider options*.
11. Discuss options for antibiotic treatment if appropriate.
12. Consider non-pharmacological and complementary therapies as appropriate.
13. Consult resident and family on all issues, ensuring informed consent for all treatment.

Liaison with pharmacist. Check *in advance* that all medications required are available in a timely manner, especially after hours and weekends.

When death is imminent

1. *Double-check* availability of next of kin (e.g., if they wish to be called any time during the night, and check that phone numbers are current).

(Continued)

(Continued)

2. Check all details on end-of-life choices (or other relevant assessment forms) to ensure resident's wishes and choices are respected and addressed (e.g., regarding hospitalisation).

3. Check resident and family requests and options for spiritual care.

4. Consider all appropriate care for family.

5. Offer resident and family support, rather than advice. Explore options to ensure that *their needs* are being met whenever possible.

6. Consider the needs of the care team.

Figure 14.2 Palliative-care checklist

Rosalie Hudson & Associates (2003); published with permission

Time should be set aside for discussion with the person and his or her family, and interpreter services should be used if necessary and available. The following aspects might be covered.

▶ Do the person and family understand the principles of palliative care?

▶ Are the person and family reassured that the nursing home or hostel is able to provide skilled and appropriate end of life care?

▶ Would the person and family appreciate written material—for example, on use of narcotics, facts about dehydration, resuscitation issues, and pastoral care services? The ready availability of written material, including current research findings, can be of great reassurance to some family members, and helps to inform their decisions as they collaborate in the planning of care.

▶ Do the person and family understand the importance of their own involvement in planning the care?

▶ Is the local doctor involved in the discussion about palliative care?

▶ Is there a need to refer to a specialist palliative-care service for medical or nursing advice?

Staff in Care Homes are well aware of the demographic changes referred to at the beginning of this chapter, and they are aware of the changing nature of residents' needs. Because there is no ready *cure* available for long-term progressive illness, so the planning of appropriate *care* is essential for the well-being of residents and their families. All of this can mean that palliative care might have to be introduced earlier rather than later, as illustrated by the story of Mrs Johnson in the Box, page 177.

Mrs Johnson

Mrs Johnson had been in the nursing home for six months. She had osteoarthritis and dementia, and a past history of breast cancer and two major strokes. She was admitted to the nursing home with decubitus ulcers over the sacral area and on both shoulders. She was malnourished, and often refused food and fluids. When Mrs Johnson had been discharged from the acute hospital, her family had been told to expect her death 'within a matter of weeks'.

In the nursing home, staff members were anxious about Mrs Johnson's increasing debility and the fact that she was in constant pain, especially when her position was being changed and her wounds were being attended. They were also unsure of the family's expectations. Although she was unable to articulate her needs, Mrs Johnson's sad eyes seemed to implore: 'Help me please'. After many weeks, when her death had not occurred as expected, Mrs Johnson's family were confused, anxious, and irritable. They said that other family priorities meant that their visiting would now need to be reduced. An atmosphere of hopelessness prevailed.

In consultation with the family and the local doctor, a palliative-care physician was called in to address the serious issue of pain management. It was agreed that Mrs Johnson's osteoarthritis and painful ulcers warranted the administration of oral slow-release morphine because milder analgesia had been tried with no effect. Within days Mrs Johnson's appetite improved. She no longer resisted every attempt to change her position. Although she had little independent movement, she readily opened her mouth to be fed.

The family's visits now increased. They provided their own roster to assist Mrs Johnson with meals whenever possible, and they brought some of her favourite foods from home. The despair previously felt by the family was now replaced by hope—not hope for a miraculous cure, but hope for improved quality of life. They were now reassured that Mrs Johnson's pain had been relieved, and they were satisfied that they were making their own contribution to her care. The palliative-care physician also explained that Mrs Johnson's death might not occur as soon as they had expected and that she might 'still have some living to do'.

As her illness took its course, Mrs Johnson became unable to swallow oral medication, and a continuous subcutaneous infusion of low-dose morphine was therefore commenced. Because it was agreed that Mrs Johnson would 'hate the indignity and invasion of a tube into her stomach', family members preferred to offer her small amounts of food and fluid as tolerated. It was now possible to give greater attention to her skin care because the nurses were no longer anxious about causing her pain. Nurses also sought expert advice on the most appropriate wound management. In spite of minimal oral intake Mrs Johnson lived for another four months.

During this time, meetings were held with the family to clarify goals and evaluate the outcome of care. All agreed that the goal was not the artificial prolongation of

(Continued)

> *(Continued)*
>
> life but the maximising of comfort. Aromatherapy, massage, music, and sunshine were added to the care plan. The family expressed their relief and satisfaction that Mrs Johnson was now so peaceful.
>
> 'She smells so nice now', observed the daughter.
>
> 'I'm sure she knows who we are and what we're saying to her', said her eldest son.
>
> 'It's taken me a long time,' said another son, 'but I've finally resolved some conflict I've had about my relationship with Mum. Visiting has now become a pleasure rather than a chore. I'm glad we've all had this extra time.'

The story of Mrs Johnson demonstrates the positive effect of introducing some aspects of palliative care—in this case, pain management—early enough to provide maximum benefit. Although Mrs Johnson's diagnoses did not readily fit the criteria for palliative care as it is commonly perceived, early and effective pain management is an essential element of palliative care, and the story of Mrs Johnson shows the increasing blurring of the boundaries between the use of palliative care in death from cancer and death from other causes. What were the options for Mrs Johnson and her family? Euthanasia? This had been mentioned by at least one family member as he expressed his frustration at seeing her suffering.

> 'Early and effective pain management is an essential element of palliative care.'

Inadequate care? Family members and staff had at first expressed concern about the quality of care, but did not know how to improve the situation. Because they believed the prognosis provided by the hospital they all thought that she would die very soon.

Entering the story

Mrs Johnson's story (Box, page 177) shows the importance of building a continuous narrative as nurses come to know the person and his or her family in their unique circumstances. It also shows how goals can shift over time. Some family members were at first reluctant to introduce palliative care: 'What's the use if she has only a few weeks left?'. Some nurses were unconvinced: 'I don't think her pain is bad enough for morphine'. The local doctor was, at first, reluctant to introduce morphine: 'I'd rather keep the morphine up my sleeve until the very end'. Given full explanations of the principles of palliative care, together with written information about the use of morphine and a comprehensive discussion with the palliative-care physician, this family not only achieved satisfaction with the care of their mother, but also received encouragement, information, and knowledge to pass on to others. 'I'm going to tell all my friends about this!' said the son who was at first the most reluctant to agree to the plan.

This story illustrates a contemporary understanding of the real nature of palliative care. Palliative care does not mean that no attempt is made to seek an improvement in health (Kellehear 1999). Rather than an excessive concentration on what might be called 'the dying trajectory', palliative care viewed in this light allows for the living of life, regardless of the expected prognosis. To enter the story of the person's life is to know and understand more clearly how the story's end might be shaped.

'To enter the story of the person's life is to know and understand more clearly how the story's end might be shaped.'

The story of Mr Papandreou (Box, below) shows how a lack of understanding of palliative care can lead to a less-than-desirable outcome.

Mr Papandreou

'What's wrong with the man in the third bed?'

'Oh, nothing much, but lately he's always complaining.'

The agency nurse looked at the chart: 'Diagnosis: Frailty. Indwelling catheter'. She wondered why Mr Papandreou had an indwelling catheter. And she wondered what a diagnosis of 'frailty' actually meant. Because the diagnosis section was undated she assumed that the data were from the date of admission. If he had been assessed as 'frail' when he was admitted four years ago, the nurse wondered about his current diagnosis!

The agency nurse continued to be concerned about Mr Papandreou's increasing distress, and she discussed the issues with some members of the regular nursing staff. In particular, she was worried about the possibility of a blocked catheter. A care attendant shook her head: 'I don't think he's got a catheter; he's never had one since I've been here, and that's three years'.

The agency nurse decided that she needed to gain a holistic understanding of this man's problems. She flicked through all Mr Papandreou's past notes and discovered a reference to osteoarthritis. Turning to the drug chart, she then noted a variety of cardiac drugs and several anti-Parkinson drugs. Did this man also have heart problems and Parkinson's disease?

(Continued)

(Continued)

'Yes, I think he's got Parkinson's', said one nurse.

'He always screams out when he is touched or turned,' observed another.

'Basically, he's a behaviour problem', said another.

The agency nurse did not say anything, but privately she was not impressed. 'I might scream if I had osteoarthritis, Parkinson's, contracted limbs, and heart problems', she thought to herself.

Mr Papandreou began to complain of severe chest pain. An ambulance was called on advice from a locum medical officer who had never met him before. Mr Papandreou died alone in the hospital emergency department.

One week later, Jim arrived for his regular Tuesday evening nursing shift. Tucked under his arm was the Greek newspaper that he always brought in each week for Mr Papandreou.

'Where's Angelos?' he asked, puzzled by the unfamiliar person in Mr Papandreou's bed.

'Oh, he's gone', said Jo, the person in the next bed.

'Where to?' asked Jim.

'I don't know,' said Jo, 'The night staff didn't say.'

The night staff knew exactly where Mr Papandreou had gone—to the hospital mortuary.

Adapted from Hudson & Richmond (2000)

The story of Mr Papandreou is that of a man whose problems did not fit the usual admission criteria for referral to a specialist palliative-care service. He had no diagnosed malignancy, and it was difficult to make an assessment of his exact prognosis. Would he have benefited from palliative care in the nursing home?

And what did Mr Papandreou think of all this? Perhaps he had decided that his multiple medical conditions could not be cured. Perhaps he assumed that his severe physical limitations meant that rehabilitation was out of the question. Because no spiritual assessment was made, it is impossible to know what life, debilitating illness, and possible death meant to him. No one had asked why Mr Papandreou's family was not involved in his care. His cultural needs were apparently 'met' by one nurse bringing him a Greek newspaper.

The last entry in his official record—'Discharged to hospital'—did not acknowledge his situation or dignify his death. The failure to communicate honestly with his room-mates showed no understanding of what it means to die in a communal environment. The goals documented in the care plan were never evaluated and, because resources were so limited, there was no debriefing or reflection on practice (Hudson & Richmond 1998).

But Jim knew . . .

The sad truth is that Jim knew, but didn't know how to respond. Jim knew that Mr Papandreou had pleaded with him, only a week ago, to make sure that he was not taken to hospital.

'I want to die here', he told Jim.

Unsure how to respond, Jim kept this to himself. He told no one until some months later.

Adapted from Hudson & Richmond (2000)

Principles of palliative care

The story of Mr Papandreou (Boxes, page 179–80) highlights the following principles of palliative care:

▶ *Choosing the site of care:* Knowing in advance whether a person has particular fears or anxieties about hospitalisation, or whether he or she prefers to be hospitalised, can have significant implications for decision making.

▶ *Staff education:* Nursing-home staff frequently deal with end-of-life issues. It is essential for staff to be educated in discussing these matters, the meaning of open communication, what cues to look for, and what to do with the information.

▶ *Staff support:* It is common for particular relationships to form between staff and residents in long-term care. Those in senior positions need to be alert to the implications this can have for staff members when a resident dies. 'Jim' (Box, above) did not have an opportunity to discuss his concerns (including his profound guilt and remorse) until many months after Mr Papandreou died.

▶ *Documentation:* Care planning for palliative care should include the person's wishes regarding crisis intervention. Although such documentation is only a guide, and although it should be regularly reviewed, wishes stated in advance can be pivotal in ensuring that agreed goals are met (Hudson 1997).

▶ *Team:* In Mr Papandreou's living and dying, 'Jim', an unqualified care attendant, held a significant place. He knew some of Mr Papandreou's unique story and might have made a valuable contribution to the team in planning Mr Papandreou's end-of-life care.

Guidelines for palliative care

Staff working in a Care Home environment usually have access to the relevant legislative framework and standards of care for dying persons. They should also have access to current guidelines for palliative care by relevant national agencies. Guidelines usually spring from a clearly articulated policy. Each organisation that formulates guidelines for end-of-life care might first consider a brief policy statement such as the following: 'Every person will have access to expert palliative care when it is considered that curative or rehabilitation goals are no longer achievable'.

The team

High-quality care is derived from *partnerships* in a team environment. This team approach includes residents and their families (or non-family carers), nursing and non-nursing staff, doctors and other health professionals, allied health specialists, and volunteers.

The role of these various team members will vary, depending on particular circumstances. For example, one person's team might include the music therapist, the chaplain, and a volunteer, whereas another person's team might include a palliative-care physician and a physiotherapist. The question that guides a team approach is: 'Who forms the team for this particular person at this particular time?'.

In nursing homes, funding constraints often determine the composition of a multi-disciplinary team—which can be less structured than it might be in a formal palliative-care service. In specialist palliative-care services the team often includes a bereavement counsellor, allied health staff, a volunteer coordinator, and a trained pastoral-care worker or chaplain. However, even if limited resources in residential care limit the provision of optimal palliative care, ingenuity and imaginative use of resources can achieve excellent results (Hudson & Richmond 2000).

Spiritual care

Although the stories of Mrs Johnson (Box, page 177) and Mr Papandreou (Box, page 179–80) do not include specific details of spiritual care, a careful reading of those stories shows that spiritual issues were at work.

The term 'spiritual issues' does not refer to these matters in the narrow religious sense (such as might be implied by the ticking of the 'religion' box on an assessment form). Nor does it necessarily mean the presence of a priest or

Dorrie's spiritual care

The term 'spiritual care' can mean different things to different people. Consider this exchange between Dorrie and a nurse.

'Dorrie, you've been talking about dying and I'm wondering if you have any concerns you would like to discuss with one of the staff or the pastoral care worker?'

'Heavens no! I've never been a religious person and I don't want any strangers visiting me.'

'If you could have your wishes met, is there anything you'd like to do in the time you have left?'

'I'd like to visit Kew Gardens and St Paul's Cathedral.'

Dorrie's nurse then arranged for Dorrie to be taken to both these favourite places two weeks before her death at the age of 99 years.

Is this spiritual care? Is it palliative care? Not perhaps in the conventional sense, but an intuitive nurse thus helped Dorrie to achieve a remarkable sense of meaning and 'closure' to her life.

Dorrie needed neither morphine nor any other particular symptom management. She was in no physical discomfort and declared that she was emotionally content. However, the nurse who recognised Dorrie's yearning to visit some familiar places one more time was contributing an essential spiritual component to Dorrie's holistic, end-of-life care.

pastoral worker in a nursing home. Rather, in this context, spiritual care encompasses the relationships and partnerships that can emerge among staff, residents, and families.

In such partnerships, issues of the meaning of life are uncovered—perhaps in fragments over time, rather than on one specific occasion. This kind of 'spiritual care' has nothing to do with an expert 'providing' care. It has more to do with carers offering to be a listening presence, and their 'tuning in' to the deeper issues of meaning confronted in each particular situation. One person's spiritual care might effectively and appropriately be addressed by the relevant chaplain or pastoral-care worker. Another person might find comfort and consolation in regular religious rituals—for example, through receiving Holy Communion, through making confession, through meditating, or through hearing familiar hymns and prayers. For others, the close tactile presence of family members and/ or trusted professional carers fills their lives with spiritual meaning. For those able to articulate their own meaning of spirituality, the invitation and encouragement can depend on a nurse's prompting, as shown in the story of Dorrie (Box, above).

Site of care

One of the pivotal questions concerning palliative care is 'site of care'. Where is the dying person's preferred place to die. Is it at home, or in hospital, or in an inpatient palliative-care unit, or in an aged-care facility? Negative stereotypes suggest the last would never be a preferred option. 'Who would *prefer* to end their days in a nursing home?' However, for a resident who feels 'at home' within a trusted environment, this might indeed be the preferred option. Is it not the unspoken thought of a person entering a nursing home: 'Will I die here? What will it be like? Will they know how to treat me? Will I suffer pain and indignity? Will I be asked what I want? Will my family have a say?'

When these questions are openly acknowledged, when fears and anxieties are identified and understood, when other options have been explored, and when appropriate care is planned, the nursing home might well be the best place in the world to die.

The question of hospitalisation also requires an individual focus, as illustrated by Mr Papandreou's story (Box, page 179–80). The life experience of Mrs Adams (Box, below) led to a different decision.

Mrs Adams

Mrs Adams had lived alone with a chronic, degenerative condition, and had required frequent hospitalisation over many years. When she could no longer care for herself at home she made her wishes quite clear after admission to the nursing home.

'If I'm ever in a position where I can't answer for myself, please take me to hospital. They have a huge file on me there. They know me well. They'll say, "Here comes Lily again" as I come through the door. And I know they'll try their hardest.'

Mrs Adams' wish was made clear in her care plan, was agreed to by her next of kin (a distant relative), and was communicated to her doctor. When the time came, as Mrs Adams herself predicted, she was transferred to hospital with a comprehensive transfer form, including her wishes. When some staff members objected that she should not have been sent to hospital to die, the authoritative, recently updated care plan was referred to.

The team had made a decision, guided by Mrs Adams' clearly stated preference.

Crisis intervention

Skilled professional nurses are able to predict, on the basis of a thorough nursing assessment, the crises that might occur in a particular person's life. For example, is the person likely to experience breathing difficulties, epileptic seizures, or haemorrhage? Has a crisis occurred in this person's recent past? How was it dealt with? How should it be dealt with next time? These are questions that are best asked within the team context, and the person and his or her family should be included in the decision-making wherever possible.

A practical outcome might be the development of a comprehensive care plan for a particular anticipated crisis. A plan might be drawn up, for example, in the event of 'severe respiratory distress'. The advice of a palliative-care physician might be helpful in this sort of example. The plan of care should include appropriate medication and adjuvant therapy, and the goal of care should be to manage the medical crisis within the nursing home, according to the wishes of the person and his or her family.

Such a plan provides excellent guidance for 'after hours' staff and agency staff who might not know the person well, and who have limited access to other team members.

Support by doctors

Dementia, chronic illness, and physical disability are the major reasons for admission to aged-care facilities, and there is an urgent need to augment current medical services with a broad range of integrated high-quality health services, including palliative-care medicine (ASGM 2001). The matter of expert medical contribution to end-of-life care is too important to leave to chance.

In their organisational and management role, nurses should ensure that visiting doctors are given every opportunity to contribute to the facility's palliative-care policies, and should ensure that medical staff are aware of agreed procedures and have access to information and resources.

In acting as advocates for residents, nurses must ensure the best medical oversight for end-of-life care.

Flexibility and review

The expressed wishes for end-of-life care are subject to change. It is impossible to predict when a person's wishes might change or when a crisis might intervene. Standards of practice and codes of conduct for professional nurses provide for professional judgment to be made at the time. When this is made clear to residents and families it provides increased confidence. It is comforting to know that skilled professional nurses will make considered, timely decisions in the best interests of the person when required. For these reasons, the best plans are always subject to flexibility and review, and are never 'written in stone'.

Death, dying, and dementia

For some people, the words 'death', 'dying', and 'dementia' have become the 'dreaded three d's'. Dying of dementia in a nursing home is often considered to be the ultimate indignity, the last resort, and the worst of all deaths. How can nurses turn this perception around, such that the community can look with confidence to nursing homes as being places in which people with dementia are accorded the utmost dignity and the best end-of-life care available?

At least 70% of nursing-home residents in England have probable clinical dementia (MacDonald et al. 2002) and this calls for skilled care based on contemporary research. End-of-life issues require compassionate understanding and insight into the specific needs of those who are confused or inarticulate. Decision-making in these circumstances is a challenge for families and staff, particularly if there is a difference of opinion (Abbey 1998).

The issues of advocacy, advance planning, flexibility, and review that have been emphasised in this chapter have particular relevance in dementia care.

© (Example only: Rosalie Hudson & Associates, 2003)

End-of-Life Choices

1. In the event of sudden crisis or health deterioration, do the resident or family have any *advance* preferences, wishes, or concerns regarding hospitalisation (e.g., not to be hospitalised, hospitalisation for diagnosis and speedy return if appropriate, full treatment in hospital)? If not known, consult resident and family at the time. Are resident and family aware of the options? Please specify:

   _____

2. Is there any legal documentation (e.g., advance directives, medical power of attorney)? Please describe:

   _____

3. Have resuscitation issues and options been explained to family? Yes/No (e.g., explain difference between Care Home and hospital in terms of available equipment, etc.) Comments:

   _____

4. In the event of *gradual deterioration* in resident's condition, are the resident and family aware of the facility's palliative-care policy with a focus on comfort measures and the treatment of all distressing symptoms? Further information needed? Please specify:

   _____

   (Continued)

(Continued)

Would the family welcome a family conference if the resident's life expectancy changes?

_____

5. What is the most important 'end-of-life' issue for the resident and family (e.g., quality of life/dignity issues)?

_____

6. Do the resident and family wish to receive services of a priest or minister? Please specify:

_____

7. For the purpose of timely reporting of changed health status or death, are current phone numbers accurate and appropriate? Details confirmed on: _____ (date)

8. In the event of sudden deterioration or death, would family wish to be notified at any time, day or night? ☐ Yes ☐ No   Give details:

_____

9. Would the resident and family care to specify one person as the spokesperson for the family, for the purpose of efficient and effective communication? Please specify:

_____

10. Following death, are there any special requirements relating to care of the body (e.g., cultural issues)?

_____

11. Following death is the body to be ☐ buried ☐ cremated. Details confirmed on: (date)

_____

12. Details of funeral director confirmed? ☐ Yes ☐ No. Comments:

_____

13. Are there any other wishes or choices related to end-of-life care that the resident or family would like to discuss (e.g., artificial feeding, other invasive treatment)?

_____

14. Do the resident or family require any counselling regarding end of life issues? Please specify:

Name of person completing this form (BLOCK LETTERS) _____

Date _____

Figure 14.3 End-of-life choices form
Rosalie Hudson & Associates (2003); published with permission

Terminal care or end-of-life care

When does palliative care become terminal care and what is the difference? The answer to this question lies in the increasingly complex area of predicting when death will occur.

As noted at the beginning of the chapter, demographic changes in Western societies have increased the length of the dying process, and 'terminal care' can become a misnomer in this context. The terms 'palliative care' and 'terminal care' can be encompassed by the term 'end-of-life' care. The issue then becomes not 'How long?', but 'How can we plan for this person's life and death'? Such planning includes raising in advance questions about expectations at the time of death.

Some facilities find an 'end-of-life choices' (or 'terminal-care wishes') form useful (see Figure 14.3, page 187). As with all such forms, the particular piece of paper is far less important than the relationship in which the questions are raised and the communication that follows.

Conclusion

Do dying persons in Care Homes need palliative care? This question can be put in other ways.

- ▶ Do dying people need to have all painful and distressing symptoms relieved, all emotional and spiritual concerns addressed?
- ▶ Should dying people be assisted to maintain maximum involvement in their own care until death occurs?
- ▶ Do dying people need the social supports and relationships derived from a caring team in a wider community of care?
- ▶ Do dying people need to have confidence in their carers, and should they be able to trust that they will receive holistic care for the remainder of their lives?

Palliative care focuses on the person who is living until death occurs. In response to the challenge implicit in Saunders' words, 'How people die remains in the memories of those who live on' (Saunders & Baines 1989), nurses are prompted to provide the best possible end-of-life care for every older person in their care, and to enjoy the professional satisfaction that follows.

Chapter 15

Care Plans

Sue Forster

Introduction

Care plans are only one part of nursing care. The total process, commonly referred to as the 'nursing process', was developed by Ida Jean Orlando in the late 1950s (Orlando 1961, 1972). This 'nursing process' is comprised of four parts:

- assessment (discussed in Chapter 2, page 11);
- planning (discussed in the present chapter);
- implementation; and
- evaluation.

Nurses must know how to formulate care plans that are 'user-friendly' and meaningful.

What are care plans?

Care plans are prescriptions for nursing care. They need to be specific and unambiguous so that the care-plan directions can be carried out explicitly, even in the absence of the original author. The use of nebulous statements such as 'short walks', 'pressure area care', or 'push fluids' should be avoided, because the reader does not know what they mean. For example, does a short walk mean 5 metres, 25 metres, or 1000 metres? All entries should, if possible, have a measurable criterion included.

The directions on a care plan should include:

▶ the person's name;
▶ identification number and/or date of birth;
▶ date of the entry;
▶ identification of the issue being addressed;
▶ person-centred objectives;
▶ clear interventions that are explicit, measurable, and definitive;
▶ dates for evaluation or review;
▶ signature, printed name, and status of the author; and
▶ dates related to any alterations or changes;

It is best if care plans are completed in consultation with the resident or his or her representative. Participatory care-planning is more likely to result in successful achievement of the desired objectives than is the implementation of dictatorial, task-focused regimens.

Care plans are dynamic documents that should be frequently reviewed, evaluated, and changed (if the objectives are not being achieved).

Care plans are, potentially, legal documents that can be used as evidence in a court of law. Care plans should therefore be precise, accurate, objective, legible, signed, and dated. They should be written in black or dark-blue ink, and should contain no obliterations or 'white-out' alterations.

Associated documents

All people involved in the development of a care plan should be aware of the assessment results that precede the care-plan phase of the nursing process. These results can be collated from:

▶ resident profiles (or life history);
▶ medical history;
▶ specific assessments;
▶ case conference details;
▶ allied health professional reports; and
▶ family or representative input.

The story of Olive (Box, page 191) provides an example of the sort of assessment data that forms the basis of a nursing care plan.

Olive

Olive, an 87-year-old widow, had recently been admitted to the dementia unit of a Care Home. Olive had been admitted because she was found wandering aimlessly around streets near her home in Birmingham, with no idea of who or where she was. It was obvious from her dishevelled appearance that Olive had been outside for some time, and that she was no longer able to look after herself.

Her past history was obtained from the members of her local community. Olive had been born, raised, and married in this community, and had lived there all her life. She had been the only girl in a family of 14 children. Her father had been a shopkeeper and her mother had died following childbirth when Olive was seven years old. Because she was the only female, she was expected to take on her mother's role and look after the family. She had received no formal education after age fourteen.

Olive had married Fred, a small businessman, when she was 18 years of age. She had given birth to five children, who had all predeceased her. Throughout her adult life she had worked to subsidise the business. During the day she had worked at the local shop, and in the evenings she had served behind the bar at the local pub. Fred had died when Olive was 64 years old.

On admission to the Care Home, Olive's medical diagnoses were listed as:

- Korsakoff's syndrome;
- congestive cardiac failure;
- osteoarthritis;
- traumatic amputation of the first three fingers of her right hand (three years previously);
- total deafness in the left ear, and limited hearing in the right ear;
- infected sores on both lower legs;
- dehydration and malnutrition; and
- incontinence of urine;

After examination and assessment the following data were identified:

- weight 47 kg; height 178 cm;
- mucous membranes pale; skin turgor markedly decreased;
- 17 suppurating lesions on the lower legs (infected flea bites);
- hearing severely impaired; no hearing aid;
- vision not impaired when wearing spectacles;
- incontinent of urine only early in the morning;
- constant pain in knees, elbows, fingers, and back;
- unable to button clothes or hold cutlery;
- refused all food and frequently stated: 'I'm not eating that muck';
- when offered fluids, stated: 'I want a real drink'; and
- continually wandered and tried to abscond, stating that she 'needed to get home to feed the dogs'.

To develop a care plan for Olive (Box, page 191), nurses need to analyse the collected data and place a priority rating on each issue requiring intervention. The most important issue should be placed first in the care plan, followed by the next most important, then the third most important, until all issues are placed in descending order of importance. If each issue is placed on a separate page, the order of priority can readily be changed to reflect revised assessments.

Nursing diagnosis or issue

Some nurses do not find benefit in formulating and utilising nursing diagnoses. They simply cite the 'issue' under review. The term 'issue' is used (rather than 'problem') because not all issues that require attention are 'problems'—for example, there are 'spiritual issues' and 'cultural issues' that are not necessarily 'problems'. The choice of a 'diagnosis-based' method or an 'issues-based' method is a matter to be decided by each aged-care facility. The policy should be noted in the facility's procedure manual.

A nursing *diagnosis* is a two-part statement. The first part of the nursing diagnosis should identify the matter requiring attention, which should be addressed with a person-centred objective. The second part should identify the clinical manifestation that led to the first matter being noted. All actions should address the second part of the nursing diagnosis. In the case of Olive (Box, page 191), six nursing diagnoses can be listed in order of priority, as shown in Table 15.1 (below).

Table 15.1 Examples of two-part nursing diagnoses

1st part of nursing diagnosis	related to	2nd part of nursing diagnosis
Unmet comfort	related to	joint pain
Unmet hygiene needs	related to	infected sores on both legs
Altered nutrition and hydration needs	related to	weight loss and dehydration
Altered communication	related to	impaired hearing
Unmet comfort needs	related to	wandering and absconding
Altered comfort	related to	urinary incontinence

Author's creation

The priority rankings are made on the basis of clinical judgment. There is no 'magical' formula that makes these judgments correct. In Olive's case, it was deemed that relieving her pain and curing her infections would make it easier to meet her nutritional and hydration needs. Next, it was decided that her psychological distress could be reduced by improving her ability to understand her new situation. The last priority was decided by default—simply because others were deemed more important.

Person-centred objectives

The use of person-centred objectives ensures that all actions are directed at meeting the person's needs, as opposed to being 'task-focused' or 'nurse-focused'. Using a person's name at the beginning of the written objective virtually guarantees that the objective will be person-centred.

> 'Using a person's name at the beginning of the written objective virtually guarantees that the objective will be person-centred.'

The first part of the nursing diagnosis should identify the matters that should be addressed in terms of person-centred objectives. When not using a nursing *diagnosis*, the objectives should address the unmet or altered needs related to the *issue* identified.

The second part of the nursing diagnosis should identify the clinical manifestation towards which all actions should be directed with a view to ameliorating or resolving the matter. When not using a nursing *diagnosis*, the identified *issue* should dictate the actions to be implemented.

Table 15.2 (below) illustrates Olive's care plan, with examples of person-centred objectives and actions to be implemented.

Table 15.2 Example of care plan

Table 15.2a Joint pain

Date	13 October
Issue to be addressed	Joint pain
Person-centred objectives	Olive will have minimal discomfort.
Actions	Encourage Olive to attend to her own ADLs as much as possible with 5-minute rest periods.
	Use a firm mattress on Olive's bed and encourage her to use high chairs with arm rests.
	Use a toilet seat raiser.
	Hot packs to joints and spine at 7 am and 7 pm.

(Continued)

Table 15.2 Example of care plan

Table 15.2a Joint pain cont.

Action *cont.*	Range-of-movement exercises to all joints following hot packs.
	Refer to physio for walking aids and any splints required.
	Encourage Olive to take frequent rest periods during the day.
	Ensure Olive does not mobilise without shoes that support the structure of her feet and have non-slip soles.
	Administer analgesics and anti-inflammatories as prescribed.
	Monitor/document painful episodes and responses to treatments.
	Signed:
	Name:
	Status:
	Date:
Evaluation/review date	21 October

Table 15.2b Hygiene and grooming

Date	13 October
Issue to be addressed	Hygiene and grooming
Person-centred objectives	Olive will be clean, dry, comfortable and appropriately groomed.
Actions	Supervise Olive's shower, grooming, and dressing daily and prn.
	Encourage self-care and praise Olive's efforts.
	Encourage rest periods during activities (take extra time).
	Wash hair twice a week (usually Wed. and Sat.).
	Refer to a podiatrist for foot care.
	Dress wounds with foam (8 am, 12 md, 4 pm, 8 pm) and prn depending on exudate.
	Document wound reappraisals.
	Administer antibiotics as prescribed.
	Signed:
	Name:
	Status:
	Date:
Evaluation/review date	21 October

Table 15.2 Example of care plan

Table 15.2c Weight loss and dehydration

Date	13 October
Issue to be addressed	Weight loss and dehydration
Person-centred objectives	Olive will be well nourished and achieve optimal hydration.
Actions	Provide lightweight crockery and cutlery for meals and drinks.
	Refer Olive to a dietitian and dentist.
	Offer food that Olive likes (e.g., pies, fresh fruit, finger foods, sandwiches).
	Offer Olive fortified drinks every hour (while awake).
	Administer vitamins and minerals as prescribed.
	Weigh Olive daily at 11 am and record.
	Maintain a fluid-balance chart.
	Signed:
	Name.
	Status:
	Date:
Evaluation/review date	21 October

Table 15.2d Impaired hearing

Date	13 October
Issue to be addressed	Impaired hearing
Person-centred objectives	Olive will achieve optimal communication.
Actions	Refer Olive to an acoustic laboratory for testing and provision of a hearing aid.
	Gain visual contact with Olive before trying to talk to her.
	Talk on her right side.
	Speak slowly, distinctly and in a normal tone (do not shout).
	Use gestures, touch, and picture cues.
	Ask Olive to repeat what was said if there is a suspicion that she did not hear.
	Signed:
	Name:
	Status:
	Date:
Evaluation/review date	21 October

Table 15.2 Example of care plan

Table 15.2e Dysfunctional behaviour (wandering and absconding)

Date	13 October
Issue to be addressed	Dysfunctional behaviour (wandering and absconding)
Person-centred objectives	Olive will have minimal distress.
Actions	Monitor/record episodes and patterns of wandering and attempts to leave the unit.
	Approach Olive in a calm and unhurried manner.
	Acknowledge her feelings.
	Walk with her and stay with her when outside the unit.
	Provide low-stimulus diversions when agitated.
	Redirect her to her room and talk to her about her dogs.
	Reassure her that her dogs are being looked after.
	Encourage her to join in with pet therapy activities.
	Ensure her light is on at night.
	Ensure her room has photos and personal items displayed.
	Signed:
	Name:
	Status:
	Date:
Evaluation/review date	21 October

Table 15.2f Urinary incontinence

Date	13 October
Issue to be addressed	Urinary incontinence
Person-centred objectives	Olive will be comfortable.
Actions	Wake Olive at 6.30 am and assist her to the toilet.
	Change bed linen and clothes when soiled.
	Clean skin after episodes of incontinence.
	Monitor Olive's toileting habits and remind her to go to the toilet before meals, rest periods, and going to bed.
	Signed:
	Name:
	Status:
	Date:
Evaluation/review date	21 October

Author's creation

Evaluation or review dates

The evaluation or review of a care plan is conducted to ascertain whether the interventions are appropriate. This is best achieved by determining if the person-centred objectives have been met. The simplest method to use when evaluating an objective is to answer the question: 'Is the clinical manifestation or issue still present?'. If the answer is 'yes', it is clear that the objective has not been met.

The evaluation procedure should be criterion-referenced, so that the results are valid and reliable. In Olive's case, her needs with respect to comfort (both physical and psychological), hygiene, nutrition, hydration, and communication should be evaluated. Depending upon the findings of the review, the actions identified on her care plan should be continued, discontinued, or changed.

Only the results of the review should be documented in a person's notes, with the actual adjustments to the interventions being written on the care plan. Duplication of data is costly in time and efficiency.

Electronic care plans

There are numerous documentation software packages on the market to assist nurses with formulating care plans. These can be efficient time-savers, and therefore of economic benefit to the organisation. In selecting a documentary software package, consideration should be given to the package's applicability to the specific facility—whether its content reflects the application of contemporary practices, and whether it meets legislative requirements.

When utilising a 'ready-made' product, it should be noted that some adjustments and inclusions might be necessary to ensure that the end result is a personalised and individualised care plan.

Hints

In writing-up care plans, nurses should be aware of the importance of choosing words that:

- respect the choice and informed consent of every person;
- ensure the dignity of every person in care; and
- avoid individual interpretation.
  For example, it is advisable to avoid the use of emotionally loaded

'Avoid emotionally loaded words that are judgmental and can be perceived as placing blame on a person.'

words such as 'uncooperative', 'aggressive', 'non-compliant', 'refused', and 'demanding'. These words are judgmental and can be perceived as placing blame on a person, or inferring that a person in care has no right to make a choice. It is preferable, simply, to document such behaviours—and leave judgment to the reader.

Similarly, an expression such as 'take for short walks' is vague and indefinite. It is better to specify the nature of the walk ('walk to the dining-room') or the distance ('walk for 50 metres'). In the same way, an expression such as 'push fluids' is vague; it is better to specify the volume of fluid ('150 millilitres') and time ('every hour').

Conclusion

Documentation associated with the nursing process has long been considered the bane of nurses' lives. This was caused by:

▶ the huge number of forms to be completed;
▶ the limited human and physical resources available to assist with the process; and
▶ the pedantic policy requirements that authors were expected to meet.

With the relaxation or abolition of rigid rules, and the adoption of 'user-friendly' documents, the negative connotations associated with documented care planning are slowly fading. Modern care plans are now formulated *with* the person, *for* the person.

Such person-centred documentation:

▶ decreases the burden of documentation;
▶ reduces the inclination to use jargon and excessive verbiage; and
▶ minimises any tendency to propose inappropriate and unacceptable actions.

Care plans should always focus on 'care provision' that emphasises the concepts of dignity and caring.

Chapter 16

Delirium and Dementia

Sandra Keppich-Arnold

Introduction

Many older people living in residential care have significant cognitive impairment. It has been estimated that the prevalence of dementia in English nursing-home residents is approximately 70% (MacDonald et al. 2002) and that the prevalence of delirium among elderly hospitalised patients is between 10% and 60% (Fick, Agostini & Inouye 2002). Delirium is thought to be unrecognised in 32–66% of patients, and delirium superimposed on dementia has been reported as occurring in 22–89% of hospitalised and community populations (Fick, Agostini & Inouye 2002).

Differentiating between dementia and delirium can be difficult, and the two can co-exist in many elderly hospital patients or nursing-home residents, with delirium often being superimposed on dementia. It is imperative that nurses identify the onset of change and document clinical observations to ensure that appropriate and timely interventions occur.

Differentiation between delirium and dementia

Detection and diagnosis of delirium are important. Patients can develop complications or die as a result of a failure to diagnose and treat a medical condition that is causing delirium—for example, a person might have an undiagnosed urinary tract infection that is causing the delirium and that also subsequently causes other significant complications. In addition, the delirium itself might cause complications—for example, inactivity as a result of delirium can lead to pneumonia and pressure ulcers, or wandering as a result of delirium can lead to falls resulting in fractures.

Although behavioural and psychological disturbances are common in dementia, it is essential to ensure that any disruptive behaviour is not due to delirium superimposed on dementia. For example, it is important to ensure that behavioural or cognitive changes in a resident with dementia are not wrongly attributed to 'sundowning' or the underlying dementing illness itself, rather than a superimposed delirium.

'It is essential to ensure that any disruptive behaviour is not due to delirium superimposed on dementia.'

Delirium usually develops over hours or days and can involve changes in a range of cognitive abilities—including memory, orientation, mood, affect, perceptions, psychomotor activity, and sleep–wake cycle. Signs and symptoms often fluctuate over short periods of time. In contrast, dementia is gradual in onset, and usually involves a progressive decline in a range of cognitive abilities—including memory, learning, orientation, attention, judgment, comprehension, language use, and calculation. This is often accompanied by alterations in personality and behaviour, which impair daily functioning, social skills, and emotional control.

Features that differentiate delirium from dementia are listed in Table 16.1 (page 201).

Nursing assessment

In making a nursing assessment of delirium and dementia, it is crucial that clinical observations are matched by appropriate nursing documentation. It is important that information is descriptive to ensure that longitudinal assessment and appropriate management are facilitated.

Table 16.1 Differentiating delirium from dementia

Feature	Delirium	Dementia
Onset	acute	insidious
Duration	hours to weeks	months to years
Course	fluctuating	progressive
Awareness	impaired	usually normal
Orientation	disorientated (especially in time)	usually impaired
Attention	inattention with poor concentration	usually normal
Perceptual changes	visual misperceptions common (fleeting and simple)	more likely to be complex and delusional (e.g., belief that someone has stolen possessions)
Thinking	slow or accelerated	impoverished and vague
Memory	recent and immediate impaired, but usually intact knowledge	recent and immediate impaired; some loss of general knowledge fragmented sleep
Sleep–wake cycle	disrupted	

Adapted from McLean (1987)

A ten-point assessment plan is recommended (Hall & Hassett 1998):
 ▶ find out from the person what he or she thinks the problem is;
 ▶ establish pre-morbid function and current function;
 ▶ understand the social and personal perspective;
 ▶ uncover the health history;
 ▶ identify the medication history;
 ▶ determine routines;
 ▶ establish level of sensory function;
 ▶ undertake cognitive and mental state assessments;
 ▶ establish cognitive patterns; and
 ▶ validate the history provided.
 Each of these is discussed below.

Find out what the person thinks the problem is

The nurse should try to obtain the information from the person or his or her family. Both the onset and the course of the changed behaviour should be established. What changes have taken place? When did they start? What effect have they had on the person's life?

Nurses and carers need to listen carefully to family members' explanations of routines. The assessment of clinical risk factors can lead to finding solutions to problems.

Ken

Ken was an 81-year-old man with a history of emphysema and heart disease who lived with his daughter. Ken's memory had deteriorated, and he had been diagnosed as suffering from vascular dementia.

Each week night he was confused. He would wake during the night talking incoherently, and was disorientated in his home environment. However, at weekends, his capacity to communicate and to manage independently improved.

A trial-and-error problem-solving approach revealed that mild dehydration was the major contributing factor. During the week Ken was at home alone during the day and looked after himself. His fluid intake at these times was poor. However, at weekends, his daughter assumed responsibility for his daily care. Under her supervision, his daily fluid intake was adequate.

The longer-term management plan therefore included provision for better support during the week. Ken was then able to optimise his fluid intake, and the episodes of week night confusion decreased.

Establish pre-morbid function and current function

Relatives might report a rapid and significant decline from pre-morbid function. Such a history indicates delirium, rather than dementia.

Nurses should assess the person's previous coping capacity. Some people have always been poor at remembering names, or at organising time and appointments. It is therefore important to recognise how function has changed and the time frame over which it has changed.

'It is important to recognise how function has changed and the time frame over which it has changed.'

Determining the rate of decline in daily living skills is also instructive. Social supports and activities are important indicators of social functioning.

Understand the social and personal perspective

Dementia compromises a person's ability to adapt to social and environmental changes. Life changes—such as the death of a spouse, loss of income, or separation from family—are all stressful events that can contribute to changes to health status. These events should be fully explored and documented.

It is important to establish patterns of alcohol intake. Alcohol intake can be underestimated or unreported unless appropriate questions are asked. It is important to quantify alcohol intake to ensure that consumption is accurately identified. Withdrawal from alcohol can induce a withdrawal syndrome and associated delirium.

Diet and dietary patterns are important. Nutritional deficiency is a contributory factor to delirium. Older people who live alone can have poor diets, and prescribed medications can alter absorption of important key nutrients.

Uncover the health history

A thorough health history can be important in discovering patterns of illness or injury that require further investigation. Urinary tract infections, chest infections, and pain are more likely to cause delirium in a person who has pre-existing dementia.

> 'Urinary tract infections, chest infections, and pain are more likely to cause delirium in a person who has pre-existing dementia.'

Some examples of questions to ask are:

▶ 'When did you last see your doctor?'
▶ 'What do you think your major health problems are?'
▶ 'What do you do to stay healthy?'
▶ 'What illnesses have you suffered in the past?'

Infection, anaemia, nutritional deficiency and a number of other conditions can contribute to confusion in elderly people. It is important to establish a clear medical history to ensure that nothing has been overlooked.

Identify the medication history

Older people tend to take more medications than younger people, and this increases the risk of delirium. It is not unusual for older people to take both prescribed and over-the-counter medications. Sometimes older people consult more than one doctor, and medications might be duplicated. Sometimes side-effects go unreported or unnoticed.

Marg

Marg was an 82-year-old woman who had been admitted to hospital with a diagnosis of dementia. Over the course of three months she had seen a number of health professionals and had been treated and managed in various parts of the healthcare system. Despite this, Marg's mental condition continued to deteriorate.

After she had been admitted to hospital, a nurse took the time to examine Marg's past medical history in detail. She noted that Marg had, for some years, been taking thyroid medication. However, this had apparently been overlooked in recent months and no one had ensured that Marg take her medication.

Recommencing the medication was not sufficient to reverse the dementia entirely, but it reduced Marg's acute confusion and allowed her to return home with appropriate care supports.

Determine routines

Many older residents have highly individualised routines. These routines include exercise, meals, entertainment, community activities, radio listening, and television viewing. Nurses should also identify personal hygiene routines, including toileting and sleep patterns.

Maintaining patterns of previous behaviour is important in adjusting to unfamiliar environments. Interruption to an established routine can undermine well-being and contribute to altered cognitive function.

Establish level of sensory function

Auditory or visual impairment can exacerbate cognitive difficulties. A hearing-impaired person might not hear a request, and might be too embarrassed to ask for clarification. The person's response might seem to be incongruous, but it might actually be an appropriate response to a misunderstood request or comment.

It is therefore important that nurses take account of possible sensory deficits in assessing cognitive function of those in their care.

Undertake cognitive and mental state assessments

Several clinical tools for assessing cognitive function have been developed, including the mini-mental state examination (Folstein, Folstein & McHugh 1976). However, the reliability of this tool to distinguish between acute and chronic conditions is not adequate, and it must be supplemented by a mental-state assessment and interview (Meagher 2001). The confusion assessment method (CAM) is useful because of its relative simplicity and reliability across a number of settings (Edlund et al. 2001).

Nancy

Nancy was 78 years old and had a history of vascular dementia. She lived in a nursing home and had become increasingly distressed as a result of apparent visual hallucinations. She described 'seeing cats'. She was particularly distressed at meal times when she saw cats climbing over the tables and across other people's meals.

A nurse performed a routine nursing assessment. During this assessment, the nurse held up her hand to ask Nancy how many fingers she could see. Nancy became distressed, and began crying. When she settled, she stated that she had actually seen a cat. Nancy was misinterpreting hands as cats. The explanation was that Nancy suffered from agnosia. She failed to recognise familiar objects.

Management strategies included removing Nancy from the dining-room for mealtimes and ensuring that nursing staff wore brightly coloured gloves during all interventions to alter her visual experience. Nancy's agnosic problems settled significantly as a result.

A positive CAM result is indicated by (Inouye 1998):

▶ the presence of acute onset or fluctuating course and inattention; and one or both of the following:

▶ disorganised thinking *and/or* altered state of consciousness.

Establish cognitive patterns

Two different subtypes of dementia have been identified—cortical and sub-cortical dementia (Cummings 1986). A recognition of dementia subtypes can be clinically useful in assessing motor and behavioural difficulties, and in planning an appropriate nursing response.

A *cortical* pattern is manifested as intellectual deterioration including problems with language, learning, perception, and calculation. Clinical observations might include:

▶ *loss of language function*, in which comprehension or expression of words is impaired; (initially this presents as difficulty in word finding, but ultimately can lead to 'word salad');

▶ *agnosia*, which is evidenced by an inability to recognise familiar faces or objects, and the inability to perform learned motor acts such as dressing and feeding;

▶ *impaired memory*, particularly in the area of new learning; (memory function might also appear worse due to language difficulties);

▶ *apraxia*, or impaired capacity to undertake learned motor skills; (this incapacity occurs despite the person being physically able and willing to complete tasks, and can lead to increased frustration due to decreased ability to self care);

▶ *impaired judgment*; and

▶ *retention of insight* (which can lead to mood changes).

A *sub-cortical* pattern of dementia results in a disturbance of fundamental functions, which affect motivation, mood, attention, and arousal.

Functional disturbances include:

▶ *psychomotor slowing*, producing stooped posture, rigid gait, and a fine tremor;

▶ *impaired memory*, in particular the ability to recall specific information; (retrieval can be aided by providing clues and allowing the 'story' to be built up over time);

▶ *affective and emotional disorders*, which are evidenced by increasing irritability or apathy (apathy can easily be mistaken for depression);

▶ *reduced or impaired problem-solving abilities*; and

▶ the presence of *bradyphrenia* (slowness of thought), and the slowing down of all mental processes; (this is often associated with repetitive behaviour, including repeating the same task over and over again).

Chris

Chris was an 82-year-old man. He had a 5-year history of dementia and was living in a nursing home. Chris had become increasingly irritable and angry at nursing staff. Personal hygiene had become a daily challenge for nursing staff.

In the nursing assessment of Chris it was recognised that he was slow to respond to all verbal questions. Sometimes, his response to a question took three minutes.

In managing his slowed mental processes, staff took time in their communications with Chris and added a number of verbal cues to visual cues. These strategies resulted in Chris comprehending what was expected of him.

Validate the history provided

By speaking to a number of people, nurses should always confirm the history that has been provided. General practitioners are often a good place to start. However, nurses should be aware that it is not uncommon for people to mask their problems and to behave appropriately when in a well-learned situation— such as their own home or the doctor's surgery.

Managing care

Establishing cause

The first consideration in care management is to first determine that the person does have a diagnosis of dementia. Once this has been established, management depends on the severity of dementia.

There are many different causes for dementia. The Box below lists some causes of dementia.

Causes of dementia

The more common causes of dementia include the following:

- dementia of the Alzheimer's type (DAT)—the most common dementia; follows a progressively deteriorating course;
- Lewy body dementia—presents as a syndrome with fluctuating cognitive impairment associated with hallucinations;
- vascular dementia—often associated with a stepwise deterioration with a medical history of stroke or hypertension;
- Pick's disease—occurs predominantly in younger people (under the age of 65 years) with relative lack of memory impairment;
- alcohol dementia—associated with prolonged excessive alcohol use; causes frontal lobe changes and short-term memory problems out of proportion to other cognitive deficits;
- Parkinson's disease—can produce subcortical dementia; bradyphrenia is a significant feature;
- Creutzfeldt–Jakob disease—a rare, but fatal, brain disorder caused by a transmissible organism; the disease is rapidly progressive with pronounced mental deterioration;
- severe head injury—can produce permanent change in a person's cognition and can influence behaviour and personality.

Adapted from McLean (1987, 1993)

Potentially reversible dementia is rare. However, it is important to optimise a person's physical health and well-being to reduce the risk of unnecessary burden of disability.

Potentially treatable causes of dementia include:

- depression;
- Parkinson's disease;
- metabolic disorders;
- alcohol-related dementia;
- subdural haematoma;
- vitamin B_{12} deficiency;

‣ drug toxicity;
‣ epilepsy;
‣ normal pressure hydrocephalus;
‣ endocrine disorders such as hypothyroidism; and
‣ exposure to heavy metals.

In contrast, delirium is almost always due to a treatable underlying cause. Recognising risk factors that contribute to the development of delirium and establishing protocols for the management of cognitive impairment can contribute to better management outcomes (Cole, Primeau & Elie 1990; Inouye & Charpentier 1996).

> 'Delirium is almost always due to a treatable underlying cause.'

People are more likely to develop delirium if they have:
‣ visual or auditory impairment;
‣ increasing age;
‣ malnutrition;
‣ physical restraints;
‣ more than three medications; and
‣ a bladder catheter in position.

The most common cause of delirium in elderly people is dehydration (Brietbart, Gibson & Tremblay 2002).

A medical emergency

Through positive care planning, it is possible to reduce the risk of delirium. However, if delirium occurs it should be noted that this is a medical emergency and requires urgent medical response. At the onset of delirium it is imperative to seek resolution through appropriate intervention.

Attention must also be provided to a person who is in the post-delirium stage. It is important to provide psychological support to people who have experienced delirium, and to talk to them about their experience.

It is also important to identify the cause of the episode of delirium, and to consider the possibility of recurrences.

Family and carers' perspective

Providing information and advice to families and carers is very important. The carers' needs must also be fully incorporated into all planned interventions. Carers should be assisted to comprehend the complex needs of the person they care for. It is essential to educate the resident's family and friends about the nature of the changes that confront them.

Family members should be encouraged to reassure and reorientate the person. They can increase the familiarity of the environment by spending time with the person and providing familiar objects.

Supportive interventions

When a person presents with cognitive impairment, it is imperative that care planning incorporates strategies to prevent the risk of delirium. A range of interventions and protocols has been suggested to manage the dementia and delirium. The Box below lists a range of suggested programs and protocols.

Supportive interventions

Orientation programs

Establishing orientation programs is important to residents. The environment should be signposted and routines should be cued to make the environment supportive and reassuring. Through the use of orienting communication, orientation boards, name badges, and daily routines established and posted for residents and carers, familiarity with the environment and daily routines is enhanced.

Sensory programs

Ensuring that people have their spectacles and hearing aids minimises sensory deprivation. Effective lighting, signage for toilets and bathrooms, and adaptive equipment are all useful tools for supporting those with sensory loss.

Exercise and activity programs

Exercise programs and activities are important for all people. Benefits include the enhancement of strength and mobility, thus reducing the risk of falls. Exercise also aids general well-being and health. It is important to avoid the use of restraint or immobilising equipment (which includes an indwelling catheter). People with cognitive impairment have a reduced ability to understand the purpose of such equipment, and this can result in increased distress and paranoid thinking.

Hydration programs

To counter the risks of dehydration it is important to ensure that fluids are available and within a person's reach. If this is not possible, it is important to offer regular fluids to achieve appropriate hydration.

Sleep protocols

Sleep patterns in residents can be problematic. It is a good idea to consider a non-pharmacological sleep protocol, which includes warm drinks, herbal teas, relaxation tapes, music, and massage. It is imperative that residential and hospital settings consider noise-reduction strategies to encourage uninterrupted sleep. This strategy might also need to include the rescheduling of medications and other nursing activities.

Adapted from O'Keefe (1999)

Conclusion

A plan for managing dementia and delirium in older people should be based upon thorough assessment. The implementation of such a plan can reduce unnecessary disability, and can achieve significant improvement in quality of life. Even though older people with underlying dementia are more vulnerable to delirium, preventative strategies can produce significant benefits.

'Nursing care for a person with dementia should be positive in outlook, preventative in strategy, and based on the individual needs of the person.'

Nursing care for a person with dementia should be positive in outlook, preventative in strategy, and based on the individual needs of the person. It is imperative to identify cognitive deficits and to manage the resulting symptoms using the nursing process.

Chapter 17

Medications

Geoff Sussman

Introduction

The ageing of the population brings with it many problems. Many of these are quite apparent, but others are less obvious. Some of the latter relate to medications and their use. Several studies have shown that medication-related illness among older people is rising. For example, adverse drug reactions are implicated in 5–17% of hospital admissions and while in hospital 6–17% of older in-patients experience adverse drug reactions (Cunningham et al. 1997, Mannesse et al. 1997, Mannesse et al. 2000).

Medication problems in older people

Several factors influence medication use and the problems experienced by ageing people in relation to the use of medication. These include:

- ▶ the ageing process and changes in the pharmacokinetics of drugs;
- ▶ polypharmacy;

▶ problems of compliance; and
▶ side-effects.
Each of these is discussed below.

The ageing process and pharmacokinetics

The major changes resulting from the process of ageing are physical changes, body composition changes, and changes in organ function.

The physical changes with ageing include alteration in weight, contour, and posture. The changes of body composition are changes in lean body mass, water, bone, and fat. Organ systems change significantly with ageing. Most organs and systems show diminished function—including the cardiovascular system, respiratory system, nervous system, digestive system, musculoskeletal system, and endocrine system. When compared with a 30-year-old male, a 75-year-old male has only 56% brain weight, 70% cardiac output at rest, 69% kidney function (as measured by glomerular filtration rate), 35% taste sensation, and 40% maximum oxygen uptake during exercise (Shock 1962).

Drugs enter the body orally, by injection, by inhalation, by infusion, or by being applied topically. The body then absorbs and distributes the drug—either as free drug or bound to plasma proteins—to the organs and tissues. Drugs are then metabolised into either *inert compounds* (that have no pharmacological activity) or into *active fractions* (that exert an effect on the body before being excreted by the kidneys, liver, lungs, and skin). These metabolic processes are altered as people age because of changes in absorption, distribution, metabolism, and excretion.

Because of changes in the pH of the stomach, delay in gastric-emptying time, and changes in gut motility, the ability of the gut to absorb drugs alters, as does the breaking-down of individual medications. Some drugs are broken down by the acid pH of the stomach to begin the process of decomposition. If this is reduced, the distribution of that drug can be affected. With ageing, the acid levels of the stomach are reduced and this can alter drug absorption. In contrast, some drugs are coated to prevent breakdown by the acid pH of the stomach and are broken down by the more alkaline pH of the small intestine. However, if the normal motility of the gut is reduced, and there is a consequent delay in gastric-emptying time, these drugs remain in the acidic stomach

'The metabolism of drugs is altered as people age because of changes in absorption, distribution, metabolism, and excretion.'

and will be broken down, thus not reaching the small intestine in time to be effective.

Medication problems in the elderly

The problems experienced by ageing people in relation to the use of medication can be summarised as follows:
- the ageing process and changes in the pharmacokinetics of drugs;
- polypharmacy;
- problems of compliance; and
- side-effects.
  Each of these is discussed in this chapter.

The level of plasma proteins in the blood also affects drug metabolism and distribution. These proteins bind drugs for transport and distribution throughout the body. Malnutrition or a poor diet reduces the level of albumin and other proteins in the blood. The consequence is that more free drug is transported, leading to a more pronounced effect of the drug and a diminution of length of action of that drug. In these circumstances, to lower the risk of an adverse reaction, it might be necessary to reduce the doses of drugs known to be highly protein bound.

Another factor that affects the activity of drugs as people age is the ability of the liver to metabolise (and thus detoxify) drugs before excretion. A reduction in hepatic blood flow, enzyme activity, and liver mass can all lower the rate of drug metabolism in the liver.

Ageing also reduces kidney function, which affects the capacity of the kidneys to eliminate free drugs or their metabolites. Hypotension and cardiac failure can also decrease kidney function. Such a reduction in the ability of the kidneys to excrete drugs and their by-products from the body might require dose reductions. The dose effect can be modified either by a reduction in dose of the drug or by increasing the time between doses.

Polypharmacy
Definition and causes
Polypharmacy can be defined as the administration of a number of drugs to a patient for the ongoing treatment and management of their conditions.

Older people tend to take a larger number of medications because of the presence of chronic diseases, misdiagnosis (due to atypical presentation of some diseases in older people), inappropriate prescribing, and use of non-prescribed medication.

Factors in producing polypharmacy

Polypharmacy is a multifactorial problem. Some of the factors playing a part in this problem include the following.

The belief that all diseases require medical treatment with drugs

Many people believe that that they are not receiving proper treatment if a drug is not prescribed for every medical complaint. Indeed, some people think that medication is the *only* way to treat most signs and symptoms.

The belief that drug therapy should be continued indefinitely

Many older people believe that a drug, once prescribed, should never be changed. For example, people who have been prescribed night sedation while in hospital might continue to use the drug indefinitely.

Visiting several different doctors, alternative therapists, and pharmacists

In seeking second opinions and alternative views, people can visit several different doctors, alternative therapists, and pharmacists. These people can end up with medications from all of these practitioners, many of whom will be unaware that other practitioners have already recommended other drugs to these older people.

Increased use of over-the-counter proprietary medicines and herbal products

The use of herbal, non-traditional, and alternative therapies is increasing as some people become disillusioned with traditional medical treatment. These products are believed to be 'natural' (and thus presumably 'safe'), and once patients commence using the products they are often reluctant to discontinue. However, there are now reports of adverse reactions to a number of herbal products—including dermatitis, bronchospasm, anaphylactic shock, haemolytic anaemia, diarrhoea, nephropathy and colitis.

Because the population is ageing, people have more chronic conditions and need more drugs to manage them. The management of these chronic diseases might not always be satisfactory, and this can prompt older people to seek advice and treatment from a number of practitioners, including non-traditional and alternative therapists, all of whom might prescribe another medication.

Part of the reason for the increase in medication usage in older people relates to the side-effect profile of many drugs. It is not uncommon for people to experience symptoms such as nausea, changes in bowel function, sedation, indigestion, and cardiac or respiratory changes. These signs and symptoms, although related to medication, can be perceived as symptoms of other diseases, and new drugs thus become added to the ones already being administered. (For more on side-effects of drug use in the elderly, see 'Side-effects', this chapter, page 218.)

There are thus many factors that contribute to the high level of polypharmacy in older persons. The Box on page 214 summarises these.

Effects of polypharmacy

The greater the number of drugs used, the greater the risks of interaction, side-effects, and adverse drug reactions.

Many drugs, when given together, will interact. These interactions can increase or decrease the activity of either or both drugs. The absorption, metabolism, and excretion of the drugs can be affected. Drug combinations can result in chemical interactions that affect the action of the drugs and result in unwanted side-effects. Some drugs can also block or enhance the receptors of other drugs resulting in an increased or decreased effect.

> 'The greater the number of drugs used, the greater the risks of interaction, side-effects, and adverse drug reactions.'

Substances such as alcohol can have a marked effect on the action of a number of drugs. Alcohol can increase a person's sensitivity to a drug, and some drugs can increase the effects of the alcohol. A number of drugs will be affected by co-administration with alcohol. Alcohol can either stimulate or inhibit the metabolism of a number of drugs. These include warfarin, methotrexate, diazepam, salicylates, phenytoin, sulphonureas (oral hypoglycaemics), nitrates, and antidepressants.

For more on side-effects, see 'Side-effects', this chapter, page 218.

Problems of compliance

Types of non-compliance

One of the essential aspects of the use of any medication is strict adherence to the directions for use of the drug. Many people do not take their medicines correctly. Table 17.1 (page 216) shows some common ways in which people do not adhere to directions.

General reasons for non-compliance

People give various reasons for non-compliance. Some simply forget to take the medication (because they slept in, were busy, were going out, and so on). In other cases, the person's symptoms have disappeared so they believe that they no longer need to take the medicine. This is a serious problem if the medication is being taken to control a chronic illness. The fact that the person is symptom-free indicates only that the medication is, in fact, performing the role for which it was prescribed.

Table 17.1 Examples of non-compliance

Non-compliant action	Examples
Not taking drugs at the specific times ordered	To ensure absorption, a medication might need to be taken before food, but the person takes it after food.
	OR
	A drug might be prescribed to be taken four times a day, but is taken only twice a day by the person.
Interrupting the treatment	Antibiotics should be taken until the course is completed. However, some people discontinue the treatment if their symptoms have improved.
Not adhering to the dose to be administered	The dose of an analgesis might be two tablets 4-hourly for pain, but some people take four tablets at a time to increase the analgesic effect.
Adding other drugs not prescribed	It is not uncommon for a person to give unused supplies of a medication to a friend who has similar symptoms to those for which the drug was prescribed.

Author's creation

Some people neglect to have the prescription re-dispensed—even when ongoing treatment is required. Some might simply forget to have the repeat prescription filled. Others might have run out of prescriptions, but choose to wait for their next doctor's appointment, rather than making a special trip. The term 'concordance' is increasingly used to describe how medication taking may be optimised through prescribers working closely with their patients. This approach acknowledges the choices and beliefs which shape individuals' medication-taking behaviour.

Some people do not comply because they experience side-effects from the medicine. Instead of speaking to their doctor, nurse, or pharmacist, some people simply cease the medication.

Age-related reasons for non-compliance

There are also some age-related factors that lead to increased non-compliance among older people. Table 17.2 (page 217) sets out some of the reasons for older people not complying with directions for taking medication.

Table 17.2 Age-related factors in non-compliance

Reason	Example
Increased age	Changes in body systems can lead to an increased risk of adverse reactions.
Changes in cognition, dementia, forgetfulness	Changes in cognition and understanding of requirements can cause difficulties with compliance.
Living alone	There is increased potential for non-compliance among those who do not have others to remind and guide them in proper taking of medication.
Confusion with drug names	Many drugs have similar names, and this can cause confusion in older people.
Complicated administration	Some people need to take a large number of drugs, with different numbers of tablets being required at different times of the day.
Size, colour, taste	Most tablets have a marked code on their surface, but it is not easy to see. People can become confused about this, and about the size and colour of the tablets that they are meant to be taking.
Packaging	Medications presented in blister packs or child-proof containers (for safety) can be difficult to open. Some 'child-proof' containers can actually be 'adult proof', especially for older patients with arthritis or reduced strength in their hands.
Visual impairment	Patients with visual impairment can find difficulty in reading the directions on the label of medication, thus increasing the risk of error.
Lack of understanding and poor patient education	If a doctor or pharmacist does not have time to make sure the person understands why and how the medication must be taken, there is increased potential for non-compliance.
Cultural or idiosyncratic factors	Some people will not do what they are asked to do. Some older people might be 'set in their ways', or have a conscientious objection to certain practices (perhaps unstated), or they might simply be people who choose not to comply with advice.

(Continued)

Table 17.2 Age-related factors in non-compliance (*Continued*)

The use of a single container for many of the person's drugs	Older people with many medications to take each day often put all their drugs into one container, especially if they are 'out and about' during the day. This can cause confusion as to which medicine to take. There is also a risk that drugs stored in an unsuitable container might become unstable.
Hoarding of drugs	Older people who have been frugal throughout their lives might have a reluctance to dispose of drugs that are out of date or no longer required because they see this as 'wastage'.

Author's creation

Side-effects

As discussed above (see 'The ageing process and pharmacokinetics', page 212), physical changes associated with ageing predispose people to a wider range of adverse drug effects and drug interactions. A number of commonly prescribed drugs can cause unpleasant and sometimes debilitating side-effects—especially in older people. Table 17.3 (page 219) presents some side-effects of drugs commonly used in older people.

Certain medications should be avoided completely in older people (WHO 1981). These include barbiturates (because of confusion), bethanidine (postural hypotension), chlorthalidone (prolonged diuresis and incontinence), nitrofurantoin (peripheral neuropathy), and phenylbutazone (aplastic anaemia, hypotension, and toxic hepatitis).

Recommendations

There are several ways in which older people's nurses can assist those in their care to prevent ill-effects from medication, or at least reduce the risks.

Reviewing drug requirements

Nurses should regularly and frequently review all medications being used to ensure that they are still needed. Medications that are not needed should be ceased, and those that are needed should be reviewed to ensure the lowest effective dose is being taken. This review should be undertaken in conjunction with the person's carer, doctor, and pharmacist.

Table 17.3 Side-effects of dugs commonly used in the elderly

Drug	Side effects	Mechanisms of action
Digoxin	Nausea and vomiting; cardiac arrhythmias; confusion; weakness; visual disturbances	Reduced excretion in older people
Diuretics	Electrolyte disturbances; higher urea and glucose; altered calcium excretion	Effects on kidney function
Antiemetics	Ataxia; extrapyramidal side-effects; increased risk of falls and dizziness	Central nervous system actions
Non-steroidal anti-inflammatory drugs (NSAIDs)	Gastrointestinal upset; oedema; cardiac failure; renal failure; confusion; bleeding tendency	Gastric irritation; fluid retention; renal impairment; central nervous system action; anti-platelet function
Hypnotics and sedatives	Dependency; excessive sedation; confusion; ataxia; increased risk of fractured neck of femur	Central nervous system action
Codeine-containing analgesics	Constipation	Reduced intestinal and gut motility

Author's creation

Nurses should ensure that their patients' diagnoses are reviewed regularly and frequently. Patients should be encouraged to speak frequently with their doctors and pharmacists about their medications—especially if there have been changes made to the drugs being used, or to the dosage schedule.

Reviewing compliance

Nurses should check their patients' knowledge of the dosage schedule of their drugs to enhance compliance. Dosage schedules should be simplified if possible—for example, doctors and pharmacists can be asked to use medications that can be administered on a once-daily basis.

If a person experiences side-effects or adverse reactions, nurses should ensure that the cause is identified to differentiate symptoms of a new condition from the side-effects of medication.

Reviewing non-prescription drugs and treatments

Nurses should ask their patients about any non-prescription medication that they might be taking in addition to prescribed medication, and should check to see if there is any risk of interaction with any prescribed drugs.

'Nurses should consider the use of non-drug treatments to improve the health of those in their care.'

Nurses should consider the use of non-drug treatments to improve the health of those in their care. Diet, exercise, relaxation methods, and so on should all form part of an holistic plan of care that takes account of non-drug alternatives.

Checking for hoarding

With older persons living in their own homes, especially those who live alone, hoarding is always a possibility. When they visit, nurses should ask to see the supply of medications and check for hoarding.

Conclusion

Drugs can be a friend or an enemy, and there are many age-specific factors that increase the risk of adverse reactions to medications in older people. It is essential that medications are used with care in this age group. Caution and knowledge are essential to the safe use of medications in older people.

'Caution and knowledge are essential to the safe use of medications in older people.'

Chapter 18

Complementary Therapies

Letitia Quirk

Introduction

The terms 'alternative', 'complementary', and 'unconventional'(among others) are applied to a wide range of nursing therapies. The *Nurse's Handbook of Alternative & Complementary Therapies* makes this observation about this terminology (NHACT 1999, p. 3):

> The terms alternative, complementary, unconventional, nontraditional, and unorthodox are used interchangeably in the media and in medical literature to denote healing practices that have not traditionally been found in Western medical practice or taught in main stream medical schools.

The preferred term for these various treatments among therapists is 'complementary'—which indicates that the therapy is incorporated within conventional regimens. This is in contrast to the term 'alternative'—which can be interpreted as meaning 'in lieu of' conventional practices (NHACT 1999).

The general public's growing acceptance of complementary therapies has led many nurses to become more aware that there is a variety of strategies that they can offer their patients. Nurses have always been at the forefront of innovative health care and many are now pursuing professional training in various therapies and providing information to other healthcare providers as to how these treatments can be used to complement traditional medical regimens.

'Nurses have always been at the forefront of innovative health care.'

Over the past decade or so there has been a worldwide trend towards the use of complementary therapies in conjunction with conventional medicine. This has resulted in an increased awareness of the preventative measures that are available for the maintenance of personal health.

Definitions

Complementary medicines include vitamin, mineral, herbal, aromatherapeutic and homoeopathic products. The Australian *Therapeutic Goods Act, 1996*, defines complementary medicine as: 'Any product for oral, dermal, rectal or inhalational use containing active substances with a complementary or traditional use associated with maintenance of health or prevention of disease'.

The term 'complementary therapy' thus encompasses a range of practices and activities that aim to restore or maintain body homeostasis. Many of these practices are specialty areas in their own right, and practitioners are required to study the subject matter in depth, be awarded qualifications, and become members of recognised associations before they can apply their skills.

'Practitioners are required to study the subject matter in depth, be awarded qualifications, and become members of recognised associations.'

Complementary therapies are primarily therapeutic in orientation, but some of them can also be recreational in focus. The range of therapeutic and recreational practices is provided in the Box on page 223.

The goals of complementary therapies

The goals of complementary therapies are:
▶ to meet the individual needs of people and to achieve individual healthcare goals;
▶ to treat specific problems within a framework of holistic care;

◗ to promote healthy behaviours, including mind–body relaxation;
◗ to provide proactive (rather than reactive) health care;
◗ to alleviate symptoms;
◗ to assist relatives to achieve quality time with loved ones; and
◗ to encourage staff members to practise holistic self-care.

Complementary therapies and recreational care activities

Complementary therapies (NHA&CT 1999)

- acupressure
- acupuncture
- aromatherapy
- art therapy
- Ayurvedic medicine
- bioelectromagnetic therapy
- biofeedback
- chiropractic
- dance therapy
- dietary and nutritional therapies
- exercises
- herbology
- homoeopathy
- hydrotherapy
- hypnosis
- imagery
- laughter therapy
- light therapy
- massage and therapeutic touch
- meditation
- megavitamin therapy
- music and sound therapy
- naturopathy
- osteopathy
- reflexology
- relaxation techniques
- self-help groups
- spiritual healing & prayer
- traditional Chinese medicine

Recreational care (adapted from Hudson 2003)

- aromatherapy

Complementary therapies and recreational care activities (*continued*)

- art and drawing
- beauty therapy
- bus trips
- carving, modelling, and sculpture
- colour therapy
- comfort therapy (soft toys)
- concerts
- cooking
- craft
- dance
- dolls
- drama
- flower therapy
- games
- gardening
- music
- outings
- pet therapy
- poetry
- reading
- reminiscence
- shopping
- swimming

Complementary therapy guidelines

Existing guidelines

Nurses who practise complementary therapies within their daily nursing routine must ensure that they stay within the policy guidelines of the organisation in which they work. Nurses must also work within the guidelines set out by professional nursing bodies and associations. They should therefore upgrade their skills continuously and ensure that they have contemporary knowledge of their chosen modality.

'Nurses should upgrade their skills continuously and ensure that they have contemporary knowledge of their chosen modality.'

To ensure that an informed decision is made regarding care, the person being treated (or the person's representative) must be given information about the therapy, along with advice regarding contraindications and expected outcomes.

New guidelines

If no policy exists in a given organisation, nurses should assist in the creation of a policy document. It is important to look at the organisation's existing vision statement, mission statement, and other relevant policy documents (for example, documentation protocols, infection-control manuals, and manual-handling guidelines). Ethics committees (if available) can assist with ethical and best-practice issues. In creating a new complementary therapy policy, the relevant concepts and criteria for complementary therapies are usually readily transferable from existing policy documents.

> 'If no policy exists in a given organisation , nurses should assist in the creation of a policy document.'

To ensure success, it is essential to form a working party to discuss issues and appropriate policies with management. Interested parties within the workplace should be invited, including nurses, physiotherapists, pharmacists, residents, and their representatives.

When writing a policy, a 'statement of principles' that sets out the philosophy of the policy document is required. Such a statement should indicate why the policy is being developed and should set out the indications and benefits of the procedures being envisaged. Examples can be obtained from nurses' registration bodies, various nursing associations (including holistic nurses' associations), professional colleges, and complementary therapy associations.

When formulating the policy, practical consideration must be given to the following areas:

▶ communicating appropriately with residents;
▶ methods for gaining written informed consent, including the provision of information regarding the therapy, protocols, contraindications, and expected outcomes;
▶ cultural, gender, and religious issues;
▶ complying with relevant legislation with respect to safety, infection control, use of chemicals, indemnity insurance, and so on;
▶ the qualifications of the service providers;
▶ accountability and responsibilities of the organisation, supervisors, and practitioners;

▶ evaluation methodologies; and

▶ documentation requirements.

Once an umbrella complementary therapy policy is ratified by the organisation, each separate therapy in use within the facility will require full procedural directions to be documented and followed.

Aromatherapy

Aromatherapy is the application of essential oils to promote well-being. However, the term 'aromatherapy' indicates only one aspect of the therapeutic use of essential oils; the oils provide much more than a pleasant aroma. Aromatherapy is used to prevent illness, as well as alleviating symptoms, both physiologically and psychologically. Therapists use the chemicals within essential oils in a variety of ways to achieve desired therapeutic outcomes and to provide a pleasant calming aroma.

'Oils provide much more than a pleasant aroma.'

An essential oil is derived by various methods of extraction from the fruits, seeds, bark, stems, flowers, roots, peel, or leaves of plants. These essential oils occur spontaneously in nature, but are extremely difficult to replicate in a laboratory. An essential oil is a complex mixture of chemical compounds, and examination of the chemical constituents of a given oil indicates its likely therapeutic properties. Research has led to an improved understanding of the complex chemical structures of essential oils, and researchers have discovered the means of uptake and utilisation of essential oils in the human body.

There are many essential oils used within older people's care, of which lavender is a common example. Because the therapeutic effects of the complex chemical constituents of essential oils can have different outcomes on different individuals, the all-pervasive burning of various oils in a care setting is therefore not recommended. Indeed, it is unethical to force a treatment on residents who have not requested it, consented to it, require it, or believe in it.

'It is unethical to force a treatment on residents who have not requested it, consented to it, require it, or believe in it.'

Nurses should therefore complete a proper resident assessment, determine the resident's care needs, determine the essential oils to be applied (and their mode of application), and obtain consent.

A qualified aromatherapist should be responsible for the prescribing and mixing of the essential oils, informing staff and residents (or their representatives) of the physical and emotional benefits of particular oils (and any contraindications), writing the care plan, supervision of the application of the oils, evaluating the outcomes of the therapy, and documenting all data.

Essential oils can be applied using a variety of methods. These include:

▶ creams;
▶ direct contact;
▶ full body baths or foot baths using salts or drops; and
▶ heated oil lamps using water or fans.

Oil lamps should be placed such that they do not affect other residents. If this is difficult other residents in the room should be consulted and a notice should be displayed outside the room to inform staff and visitors.

Thelma

Thelma had been a complementary therapist who practised in reflexology and herbal medicine before her admission into a Care Home. Following her admission it was noted that she was not responding to conventional medical treatment. In particular, Thelma's behaviour was causing the nursing staff some concerns, and Thelma's husband requested the use of essential oils to address his wife's behavioural problems.

Written consent was gained from Thelma's husband and a discussion was held with her medical practitioner.

The essential oils chosen were lavender, marjoram, patchouli, and vetiver. These oils were placed into a cream base and applied to her whole body after showering, to her sacral area and hands after being toileted, and to her forehead on settling at night and when she was being attended during the night.

Thelma's lifestyle and behaviour began to improve slowly. Over the next few months she began to participate in activities around the nursing home, to interact and laugh appropriately with staff and other residents (although she was unable to speak), and to go on outings with her husband. Family members enjoyed having their mother at home for Christmas and seeing her attempt to complete some domestic chores.

The therapies improved Thelma's quality of life and her husband visited more often—often commenting on how delighted he was with her improved condition.

Reflexology

Reflexology is a practice that is thousands of years old. It has been used through the ages by many peoples since the Egyptians and Chinese first began using it around 2500 BC. Later it was practised by the native peoples of North America and by Europeans.

Reflexology is a non-invasive simple holistic technique that affects several vital body systems, including the nervous, circulatory, and lymphatic systems. Stimulating or sedating pressure is applied to the person's hands, feet, or ears, and the relaxation response and the effect of touch are thought to have an effect.

Reflexology is based on the theory that there are ten longitudinal 'zones' running the length of the body, feet, and hands and five horizontal zones running across the body. According to the theory, reflex points of the feet, hand, or ears correspond to (and can therapeutically affect) various organs and glands of the body. Congestion or tension in any part of the zone affects the entire zone. For example, the top of the big toe is said to be a reflex point for the brain, and the arch area of the foot is said to correspond to the thoracic spine and thoracic musculature.

'Some nurses provide reflexology in preference to sedatives to older people.'

Some practitioners believe that these points follow the same meridians used in acupuncture. Some nurses provide reflexology in preference to sedatives to older people.

In providing reflexology, nurses should first complete a full nursing assessment, and determine the person's care needs. Formal consent should be obtained. The person should be toileted before the session, and should then be positioned on the bed with the knees slightly bent and the feet over the end of the bed in a comfortable position. Massage tables can be used only for suitable residents. The person should be covered and kept comfortable, and his or her body and facial language should be observed carefully for reactions during and after the session.

A qualified reflexologist will be responsible for providing the therapy and for privacy, dignity, security, and confidentiality. The therapist should discuss all aspects of the treatment with staff and residents (or their representatives), including the physical and emotional benefits of reflexology. The therapist is also responsible for writing the care plan, evaluating the outcomes of therapy, and documenting all data.

Massage therapy

Many people, from the very young to the very old, enjoy a massage. Massage provides a nurturing touch that an older person might not have received in

---

Fred

Fred was a 90-year-old man with insulin-dependent diabetes who had been admitted to residential care following an above-knee amputation of the left leg. He was becoming increasingly depressed as a result of severe 'phantom pains', which various treatments had failed to alleviate.

Fred's doctor and family were informed of the potential benefits of reflexology, and consent to proceed with this form of treatment was obtained from all parties. The reflexology sessions focused on (but were not limited to) reducing Fred's pain. Fred received reflexology every three days for two weeks, and the program was then reviewed. The reflexologist played music during the sessions.

During the first session Fred felt warm sensations in his right leg with tingling in his toes and relief of the 'phantom pain' in his left leg. He was asleep by the end of the session. In view of his diabetes, blood glucose was recorded before and after each session.

Before the second session Fred asked how he could help himself to 'keep the pain away'. He was shown two points to 'work' himself, morning and night. Fred's son was keen to help and learnt how to use reflexology points while visiting his father. With each session, Fred's pain gradually subsided. By the end of six sessions Fred was pain free, apart from occasional twinges which he was able to relieve himself.

Fred stayed on a weekly program for the next three months, and was then reduced to a monthly program. It was also noted that his insulin requirements had been reduced, and that his episodes of constipation were less frequent.

---

recent times because of life circumstances—for example, as a result of the death of a spouse or separation from other family members.

Nurses frequently use 'task touch' when caring for older people—for example, during showering, toileting, or other nursing tasks. In addition to these 'task touches', nurses can use 'therapeutic touch' in the form of massage. Being held or being touched can be considered basic human needs.

Massage is the manipulation of soft tissue. It can be used to promote relaxation, to aid circulation, and to relieve pain and discomfort. Older people are often unable to tolerate 'heavy' or hard massage, and a light massage gently applied over a short period of time is therefore more appropriate in most circumstances.

Certain precautions should be observed before conducting massage therapy. Massages should be avoided in:

▶ acute inflammatory condition (because massage can intensify the inflammation);
▶ acute infectious conditions;

- ❯ circularly disorders (for example, varicose veins, phlebitis, thrombosis, embolism, aneurysm);
- ❯ the period immediately after administration of analgesic medication (because the drug can distort the person's ability to identify any discomfort from the massage);
- ❯ osteoporosis (because fractures can result from the pressure that is exerted during massage); and
- ❯ any person who does not like or wish to be touched.

In the case of any person with a post-operative condition, cancer, diabetes, recent stroke, or recent myocardial infarction, nurses should always seek permission from the person's medical practitioner and representative.

A useful massage technique for the hands and wrists begins by resting the person's hand in one hand of the therapist and gently applying cream or oil to the back of the person's hand. Using the side of his or her thumb, the therapist then gently rubs between the person's metacarpal bones from the knuckle towards the wrist. Then, using thumb and forefinger, the therapist gently works in a circular motion from the person's fingertip to the base of each finger, including the thumb.

The person's hand is then gently turned over. Cream or oil is then applied to the person's palm with the therapist using both of his or her thumbs in an outward 'fan' motion, gently stretching the person's palm.

Gentle pressure is then applied with the therapist's thumb to the fleshy pad at the base of the person's thumb while simultaneously pressing with the forefinger at the webbing at the base of the joint between the thumb and forefinger on the plantar (palm) surface.

The therapist then interlaces his or her fingers between the fingers of the person, and gently bends the person's wrist in a flexion/extension movement.

Each finger is then gently pulled and 'stretched', before rubbing across each of the person's fingernails with the pad of the therapist's thumb.

Conclusion

Although there are scientifically validated studies that demonstrate the therapeutic value of complementary therapies, nurses have different opinions on the benefits of complementary therapies. These therapies do require more time to administer, and they can take longer than conventional treatments to be effective. However, through education and practice, a new paradigm of care that includes complementary therapies will be developed and accepted into nursing.

This will require many skilled nurses and therapists working collaboratively in a multidisciplinary team. Planning and evaluation are essential in ensuring that positive outcomes are achieved. Education, research, and open and honest communication with all those who care for older people are also essential.

'A new paradigm of care that includes complementary therapies will be developed and accepted into nursing.'

The application of the organisation's policies with respect to documentation will ensure that accurate records are maintained, and will provide the necessary information for future research. Staff members who have an active role in complementary treatments should be encouraged to develop, write, and review guidelines.

Although there is a growing acceptance of complementary therapies among the general public, the evidence-based research to support such therapies in professional nursing is being developed more slowly. Nevertheless, the capable hands, hearts, and minds of nurses and therapists have achieved significant success and inspiration to their colleagues through their dedication to their chosen modalities of care.

Chapter 19

Cultural Differences

Alex Yui-huen Kwan

Introduction

> Old people need to have their feelings of self reinforced by those around
> them; the care that they are given must contribute to their independence
> against all the odds; those caring for them need all the help and support
> that they can get, if they are to act on these principles.

Dartington (1980, p. 13)

Nurses who care for people from a cultural background different from their own
should recognise that certain characteristics are ascribed to people simply by
virtue of their being identified with a particular ethnic group. In addition, for
those from a different cultural background, having a particular 'ethnic status'
carries with it a certain world view and a culturally generated complex of values
that are different from those of mainstream populations. These two aspects of
ethnicity—characteristics that are *ascribed* to people and characteristics *developed*
within the cultural group—involve adjustment problems in old age in addition
to those that are implied by the ageing process itself.

Furthermore, culturally derived stereotypes can make it more difficult for some people to access supportive services when they are needed, and this can mean that even greater hardships can be faced by various subpopulations of older people. For example, it should not be assumed that older people from minority ethnic groups will always be supported within an extended family; culturally appropriate services may still be required.

These values and world views—some overt, others hidden—can affect relationships between nurses and older people. If they are to accommodate cultural differences, nurses and carers must recognise that such values, as much as health beliefs, can influence the quality of care that they provide to older persons from different cultural backgrounds.

Cultural factors in ageing

The concept of 'culture' dates back only to the nineteenth century when, following the colonial expansion of Europe, the term was used to convey the obvious differences in the ways that people did things in different parts of the world. Originally, 'culture' meant 'tradition'—a complex set of customs. However, more recently, the term has been used to indicate the ways in which people go about daily life.

Ageing is a universal experience. However, growing older is part of the unique progression of each individual, and every person ages in his or her own way. These variations among older people dramatically increase when cultural differences are superimposed upon them. A 'normal' occurrence in one culture might be quite strange, or even deviant, in another culture. Nurses need to be aware of shared cultural characteristics within certain groups. However, awareness of similarities within a given ethnic group should not blind the nurse to the uniqueness of the individual person.

'Awareness of similarities within a given ethnic group should not blind the nurse to the uniqueness of the individual person.'

Nurses should also be aware of language difficulties. Some older people might not be able to read or write—in English or in their own language. Written messages or instructions from the nurse and health team might be misunderstood or neglected, and must often be supplemented with spoken instructions. However, because some people do not speak or understand English, the interpretation of verbal messages can also present problems. Differences in intonation, pronunciation, and sentence structure can mean that people who can *speak* English might have trouble *understanding* it when listening to others. Nurses should become familiar with the idioms, colloquial expressions, and body language that are used by the older people with whom they work. For example, an older person who does not understand a verbal or written message might nod in agreement to avoid further embarrassment. In some cases, the person might withdraw and avoid interaction with nurses.

Ethnic group experiences influence older people, and these must be considered by nurses. For example, a certain degree of ethnic rivalry exists between certain groups, and this can affect the views of older people. In addition, when people age in a foreign culture they retain some features of their own culture and acquire some characteristics of the host culture. Nurses should be sensitive to these sorts of factors, and nursing goals and interventions should take these matters into consideration.

Retaining ethnic group identification can provide support and comfort to an older person, and nurses should try to facilitate this by respecting the significance of cultural differences in their practice.

'Retaining ethnic group identification can provide support and comfort to an older person.'

Health-related cultural contexts

Health beliefs vary widely, and different cultural and ethnic groups often have quite distinct beliefs. But no social or cultural group is homogeneous. Within every group, some people know more about health, or are more interested in the subject than do other people. Some people can change their behaviour with respect to illness more readily and easily than they change underlying beliefs. For example, some people tend to be pragmatic about treatment, seeking and using anything that provides relief, while simultaneously maintaining their traditional beliefs about the causes and specific nature of their illness.

When a person's values with respect to health and illness are not congruent with the mainstream biomedical beliefs and practice, the relationship between nurses and those in their care can become fraught with difficulties. Miscommunication, incomprehension, and non-compliance can result (Fineman 1991).

Communication problems (1)

Potential for cultural misunderstanding can occur in many situations. The following example illustrates the point.

An 82-year-old Chinese woman who had been admitted to hospital with pulmonary tuberculosis became convinced that her family did not care about her recovery or welfare. She noted that her relatives came one at a time to visit her, and that they stayed for only a few minutes. In addition, the flowers and food that her family brought were immediately removed by the nurses.

The woman did not understand that Western staff members, in treating a person with tuberculosis, place high value on sterility, order, and quiet to achieve healing, and attempt to keep the person relatively isolated to decrease the risk of cross-infection.

Beliefs and values about health and illness are usually acquired early in life, and are often tenacious. In old age, many people still have the understanding of illness and treatment options that were prevalent when they were young. This can create an unrecognised 'generation gap' between older people and nurses—because nurses are frequently much younger and more recently educated than the people they care for. This generation gap is compounded when a nurse cares for older people from ethnic groups different from their own.

> 'Beliefs and values about health and illness are usually acquired early in life, and are often tenacious.'

Communication problems (2)

An 83-year-old Hong Kong man was hospitalised with metastatic prostate cancer. Because of the poor prognosis, the staff asked the family to impart the bad news. However, the idea was rejected by the family as a result of their respect for the Chinese concepts of 'saving face' and 'filial piety'.

The family members believed that it was the staff's responsibility to inform the man. In their view, because the doctors and nurses had made the diagnosis, *they* should inform the venerable old man.

Needs of older people

Contrary to common misconceptions, older people have the same needs as everyone else. Most want independence, status, health, a chance to be useful, and kind, patient friends. They want to be able to help when others need assistance—in fact, most older people much prefer to be able to help others than to have others help them.

Like other people, older people want to make their own decisions. They want economic security and they want pleasant family relationships, but they do not necessarily want to live with the family.

Nurses who care for older people need to be aware of these factors, and should strive for thoughtfulness, tolerance, patience, tact, interest, friendliness, persuasiveness, flexibility, and understanding in their dealings with older people. They should avoid pity, condescension, and impatience.

> 'Nurses should avoid pity, condescension, and impatience.'

Managing different behaviours
General comments

Older people with different cultural backgrounds often find it difficult to communicate their strong feelings directly. Many choose to deny and suppress their feelings of loneliness, frustration, and depression. They might be told that expressing feelings is childish—and thus learn to suppress feelings rather than express them.

In addition to cultural inhibitions, neurological damage, muscular weakness, and injuries can make direct verbal communication difficult.

When uncertain and unskilled at direct expression, older people often express feelings indirectly. Frustrations and fears can be expressed by grumbling about roommates and meals. Sadness sometimes motivates aimless, distracted wandering. Angry people often strike out, tease, bump wheelchairs, or are coldly silent.

For the nurse, understanding behaviour is a crucial aspect of comprehensive care of older people from different cultures. In particular, nurses should be aware of the following situations that require special understanding:

> 'Understanding behaviour is a crucial aspect of comprehensive care of older people from different cultures.'

- recently arrived residents;
- anxious people;
- depressed people;
- suicidal people; and
- angry people.

Each of these is discussed below.

Chinese cultural customs and beliefs

Chinese people are nurtured with an attitude that puts a high value on family relationships within a Confucian philosophy of an accepted 'order' to every human relationship. This 'order' refers to the line of authority, the functional role of each family member, and the place of ritual.

In a traditional Chinese family, elders and men are empowered with authority. They are leaders and spokesmen according to the 'order'. These positions are always accorded respect and prestige, and the seniors in these positions are entitled to exercise power over younger family members.

Foods are classified as 'hot' or 'cold', and a proper balance is required to maintain health. Illnesses and treatments are also classified as 'hot' and 'cold'. Many Chinese elders are particularly careful about the foods that they eat when they are sick, and avoid 'raw' foods (such as salads).

It is believed that illness can be caused by a range of factors, including:

- a disharmony of body elements (for example, an excess of 'hot' or 'cold' foods);
- moral retribution by ancestors or deities (for misdeeds or negligence);
- cosmic disharmony (for example, when the combination of a person's year of birth, month of birth, day of birth, and time of birth—the 'eight characters'—clash with those of someone else in their family;
- the interference of evil forces (such as malevolent ghosts and spirits or impersonal evil forces); and
- poor 'Fung Shui' (that is, the impact of the natural and built environment on the fortune and well-being of inhabitants).

Organs are associated with various emotions and symbolic functions. For example:

- the lungs are associated with worry;
- the gallbladder and liver are associated with anger;
- the heart is associated with happiness;
- the kidneys are associated with fear; and
- the spleen is associated with desire.

Buddhist teachings and Confucian tradition emphasise 'face' or dignity. An individual's wrongdoing causes their immediate family to 'lose face'. Older people sometimes do not admit to health problems, especially mental-health problems, because such a problem can bring shame upon their family.

A lack of eye contact, shyness, and passivity are cultural Chinese norms, and are not necessarily a sign of emotional disturbance. Many Chinese people do not want to talk to outsiders about their problems—especially psychosocial problems. Many consider that saying 'No' is impolite. This means that they sometimes go to considerable lengths to avoid saying the word 'No'. In some cases a nurse's assertiveness might be interpreted as aggressiveness or hostility.

Recently arrived residents

Nurses should learn to pronounce the resident's name correctly, and determine what language and dialect the person would like to speak. The person should be offered the opportunity to use an interpreter (preferably of the same gender). If possible, nurses should avoid using family members as interpreters because the resident might have different beliefs from those of family members. The resident might hold traditional beliefs, or might follow both traditional and modern Western biomedical beliefs, or might be in the process of integrating two cultures.

Nurses should try to elicit the resident's own understanding of his or her illness, by listening to the person's explanation of the illness—even when it seems unusual. The use of jargon should be avoided.

Family members should be involved in discussions and the development of the care plan. The resident should be invited to let staff know if staff members say or do something that upsets the person.

Anxious people

Anxiety is an unpleasant feeling of apprehension, helplessness, and uncertainty that makes thinking and acting difficult. Older people do not usually describe their problem as 'anxiety'—but rather as 'not feeling right', 'having no energy', or 'feeling nervous'. The following nursing observations can indicate anxiety in older people:

- frequently removing themselves from general interaction in the institution, becoming less verbal, appearing forlorn, and avoidance of direct eye contact;
- rapid changes of mood, restlessness, chain-smoking, and various nervous mannerisms;
- episodes of crying, demanding, and shouting when attention cannot be gained in a more normal fashion;
- irritability and taking offence easily;
- rapid pulse and respiratory rates; elevated blood pressure;
- frequent and urgent urination and, less frequently, diarrhoea;
- disturbed sleep patterns, and requests for tranquillisers or sleeping medication; and
- disturbed eating habits, (loss of appetite or overeating).

When an older person can talk about his or her anxiety and acknowledge its presence, nurses should affirm that they recognise the resident's feelings. This affirmation is supportive to the person and opens the way for further discussion. If an older person denies anxiety, or is unwilling or unable to express concerns, the matter should not be discussed further. Pursuing the issue can increase the person's anxiety.

Depressed people

A depressed person might appear sad, but not necessarily so. The person's body might seem to 'droop', he or she might walk more slowly (if at all), and the person might have slower responses to speech and other stimuli. Crying is common, and the person might clutch at nurses or other people in an attempt to relate to others.

In more severe depression, the older person might withdraw and refuse to talk to, or look directly at, other people. Dress and personal hygiene might be neglected, and meals might be skipped or food intake greatly reduced.

Nurses should not be critical during this time and should reduce any demands on the person—additional stress can worsen the situation. However, personal hygiene should be attended to, and assistance should be provided at this time. Any effort should be praised and improvement noted continually. Diversional activities and increased social contacts help such people to feel more positive about themselves and the future.

> 'Nurses should not be critical and should reduce any demands on the person.'

Suicidal people

When older people are depressed, nurses or carers should evaluate the possibility of suicide. The following factors can help to determine whether the person is in danger of self-harm.

Nurses should ask themselves the following questions:

▶ Is the resident deeply depressed?
▶ Is this depression a normal reaction to a crisis, or a series of crises, or is it a true psychosis?
▶ Has the person attempted suicide previously? Was it a serious attempt?
▶ Does the depressed resident have any support from others?

Nurses might also observe:

▶ a disturbance in the resident's sleep pattern, with early awakening in a mood of deep depression; and
▶ the resident giving away articles that were prized and not ordinarily casually exchanged.

Nurses who are very familiar with particular residents might notice subtle changes in the person that the nurse has difficulty in describing. Nurses should never ignore their feelings that something is 'not quite right'.

> 'Nurses should never ignore their feelings that something is "not quite right".'

Depressed people usually demonstrate low self-esteem and are often unable to recognise and/or accept the events that precipitated the depression. Nurses play an important role in helping the person to recognise and accept the causes of the depression and in helping the person to improve his or her self-image.

In assisting potentially suicidal persons, nurses should:

- establish rapport and trust so that the person feels comfortable in discussing problems;
- explore with the person the events that made former coping mechanisms no longer effective (a nurse's empathetic listening to past events helps the person realise that he or she still has worth);
- comment on the person's positive attributes, using sincere praise to reinforce the person's self-esteem;
- encourage and reinforce a realistic view of the person's situation;
- encourage the person to participate in group activities;
- assist family members to understand the person's behaviour and seek their cooperation; and
- try not to discourage family visits, even if this is a contributing factor to the person's depression; (nurses should try to help the two parties to understand each other and assist them in keeping communication open).

Angry people

Anger is a response to frustration and an inability to meet basic needs. Anger in older people is often rooted in feelings of helplessness. In a rage, people can strike out and express undirected anger. They often blame others, but it is usually unclear as to what should be done. Those who are blamed find themselves under attack and often feel the need to defend themselves. In these circumstances, the ability to accept of a person's anger is an important skill. In understanding anger, nurses and carers can learn about others, identify conflicts, and solve problems.

In attempting to resolve conflict with older residents, nurses should:

- develop a cooperative approach in which both persons recognise that they have contributed and should help to resolve the conflict;
- avoid trying to prove that one person is right and the other is wrong;

- demonstrate acceptance of each other as persons;
- identify and solve the underlying problem; and
- discuss how the relationship has been strengthened and hurt, and how each person has learnt about himself or herself, the relationship, and the conflict.

Conclusion

Older people, regardless of cultural differences, have varying needs. Some remain vigorous, alert, and connected with friends and relatives. Others do not have these resources, and require assistance. They might merely need medical supervision, or assistance with some activities of daily living, or extensive care because they are too weak and confused to care for themselves. They also have varying emotional and social needs, and can become isolated, depressed, or angry for prolonged periods.

All of these matters can be made more difficult if cultural differences are superimposed on the universal experiences of ageing. To provide effective care for such people, nurses need to reach out to older people, be aware of their psychological and cultural difficulties, and help them to maintain a sense of well-being in a foreign culture.

Nurses should be sensitive and helpful, seek to know older residents as individuals, and establish cooperative social situations for this group of vulnerable people.

Chapter 20

Occupational Health and Safety

Sue Forster and Wendy Thompson

Introduction

The management of occupational health and safety requires constant attention in all industries and workplaces. However, the need to apply safety-management systems in Care Homes has only recently come to prominence. This has been brought about by the requirements of industry accreditation, spiralling workers' compensation costs, and the provisions of government legislation. All industries and workplaces must achieve their respective industry standards and comply with legislative requirements. The Care Home sector is no exception.

A comprehensive and sustainable safety-management system is not only mandatory, but also judicious. The majority of residents in Care Homes can be classified as being 'at risk', and facilities who care for them have a responsibility to implement a system that will prevent these people from coming to harm. Loss of memory, disorientation, dementia, physical frailty, and sensory impairment all present risks to personal safety. Constant vigilance, supervision, assistance, and changes to the environment are all issues that should be considered in any Care Home safety-management system.

Specific occupational health-and-safety legislation requires both employers and employees to provide and maintain a safe workplace and safe work systems. Similarly, a safety-management system is not just about quick fixes, or simple expediency. It requires more than isolated activities such as monthly meetings, audits, and data collection. A safety-management system requires the development of structured systems that are based on sound risk-management principles and supported by management. Time and effort must be spent in anticipating what might happen, and then implementing risk-reduction measures into a safety-management system.

Employers and senior members of staff must recognise that health-and-safety management has the potential to reduce the organisation's exposure to injury, property damage, and financial loss.

The Health and Safety at Work Act 1974

Under Section 2 of the Act, employers have obligations to:
1. Provide and maintain equipment and systems of work that are safe and without risks to health.
2. Ensure that the use, handling, storage and transport of articles and substances is safe and without risk.
3. Provide information, instruction, training and supervision to ensure that employees carry out their jobs safely.
4. Keep the workplace environment safe and healthy.
5. Prepare and keep up to date a written safety policy, supported by information on the organisation and arrangements for carrying out the policy. The safety policy has to be brought to the notice of employees.
6. Consult with any safety representatives appointed by trade unions.
7. Establish a safety committee if requested by two or more safety representatives.

Under Sections 7 and 8, employees' duties state that, whilst at work, every employee must take care of the health and safety of himself and of other persons who may be affected by his acts or omissions.

Employees duties are qualified by the phrases 'so far as is reasonably practicable' and 'best practicable means'.

Self-regulation

A proactive policy of self-regulation is preferable to a reactive compliance with legislation. The sequence of events in developing such a policy proceeds in the following steps:

▶ information;
▶ education;
▶ audit;
▶ direction (and, if necessary, prosecution).

The first step—provision of information to all stakeholders—is the linchpin of implementing a system in an organisation. Letting people know what the plan is, when it is to be implemented, and how it is going to be put in place facilitates input into the process and reduces resistance. Imparting information should be followed by the second step—extensive and continuous education. The third phase in self-regulation involves regular auditing of all system components. As a last resort, official directions of a disciplinary nature (and perhaps prosecutions) might be required.

> 'Provision of information to all stakeholders is the linchpin of implementing a system.'

Components of a safety-management system

Safety in the workplace is the responsibility of all members of staff, residents, representatives, visitors, volunteers, contractors, and subcontractors. Everyone in the organisation should be encouraged and empowered to report hazards, risks, accidents, incidents, and potential incidents.

> 'Safety in the workplace is the responsibility of all.'

Many older people's services already have safety-management systems in place. If so, these systems should be revisited with a view to ensuring that legislative requirements are being met, and that all risks have been identified and are being addressed with appropriate risk-management policies. In other cases, a safety-management system will be developed as a new policy.

The steps in the development and maintenance of a safety-management system are listed in the Box on page 246. These steps are discussed below.

Developing a safety-management system

The steps in the development and maintenance of a safety-management system include:

- assigning members to a safety committee;
- deciding on the committee structure and nominating or electing team leaders;
- developing the terms of reference;
- developing committee meeting rules;
- holding regular and frequent meetings;
- formulating policies, procedures, and protocols;
- collecting and collating data regularly and frequently;
- discussing and debating issues raised at meetings;
- supervising the implementation of changed procedures;
- evaluating outcomes;
- undertaking statistical analyses;
- documenting all information; and
- adhering to reporting mechanisms.

Each of these is discussed in this chapter.

Assigning members to a safety committee

It is imperative that senior management actively participates in the committee and that the team leaders have the appropriate skill mix and expertise to make decisions and coordinate their teams. All members must be interested in the process and be willing to contribute actively.

Deciding on the committee structure

Many older people's services already have several committees operating in areas related to health and safety. These might include committees for quality control, infection control, medication safety, and continence management. An effective and efficient way of managing these independent committees is to link them together into one committee. This integrated approach encourages coordination and promotes a forum for active participation by all those with skills and expertise in the area of health and safety.

'An integrated approach encourages coordination and promotes a forum for active participation by all.'

Within the committee structure several teams can be formed. Smaller organisations might elect to have only three teams (such as a safety team, a clinical-care team, and a quality team), whereas larger organisations might have more teams. Each team should elect a team leader and all staff members should be encouraged to nominate a team with which they would like to be associated.

Developing the terms of reference

Terms of reference should be developed by the committee, and these should be dated and signed by the chair, secretary, and committee members. The terms of reference should include the following:
▶ the name of the committee;
▶ the composition of the committee and its teams;
▶ the roles of the chairperson and secretary, who is to fill these roles, and whether these positions are to be rotated (and how often);
▶ the purpose and objectives of the committee;
▶ the quorum required for a meeting to progress;
▶ the venue, frequency, and length of meetings;
▶ the location and time for display or circulation of the minutes and the agenda;
▶ confidentiality issues; and
▶ the requirements of proxy nominees (if any).

Developing committee meeting rules

These can vary according to the requirements of the committee. Examples of matters that should be decided include:
▶ apologies and introduction of proxy members (if any);
▶ reading of minutes of previous meeting;
▶ reading of agenda items at beginning of meeting;
▶ starting and ending times; and
▶ rules of discussion and debate.

Holding regular and frequent meetings

Initially meetings might be convened weekly to ensure that all the necessary substructure or 'ground-rules' are in place. Following this initial implementation phase, the committee should conduct meetings at least monthly (or perhaps every three months).

Formulating policies, procedures, and protocols

The safety committee should make recommendations to senior management regarding pertinent policies, procedures, and protocols that it believes should be ratified. Depending upon the committee's terms of reference, it might be expected that the committee will submit draft documents on various subjects to senior management.

Collecting and collating data

Minimal data that should be collected and collated include:

▶ identified hazards and risks;

▶ incidents, accidents, and potential incidents;

▶ compliments, comments, and complaints;

▶ audit results; and

▶ education records (attendance, induction, and competence of staff members).

A central location for the collection of data is required. The data are then logged on receipt and distributed to the appropriate team leader for further action.

Discussing and debating issues raised at meetings

Collated data should be presented to the safety committee members before their scheduled meeting so that members come prepared to discuss and debate the issues. Pre-reading and preparation prevents time-wasting and facilitates decision-making.

Supervising the implementation of changed procedures

Once an issue has been discussed and a solution has been recommended, it is essential that the proposed solution be trialled before being adopted. The trial must be supervised and evaluated. The safety committee is responsible for ensuring that the recommended actions are initiated, supervised, monitored, documented, and completed. To achieve this, members must take a 'system perspective' and be aware of the 'bigger picture'. Any change in one area of the organisation will directly or indirectly influence all other areas of the facility. For example, in an attempt to prevent falls, the committee might recommend a change in the time of assisting residents out of bed in the morning. This recommendation might affect breakfast catering, nursing rosters, laundry loads, and the commencement of cleaning and outside maintenance.

> 'Any change in one area of the organisation will directly or indirectly influence all other areas of the facility.'

Evaluating outcomes

At the completion of any trial an audit should be conducted. For example, an audit of the number of falls since the change in morning arrangements should be undertaken to ascertain whether the actions were successful.

Undertaking statistical analyses

Keeping records of all hazards, risks, incidents, accidents, potential incidents, and audit results involves the gathering of statistics. Statistics are useful only if they are analysed. Comparing and contrasting data over a period of time is useful in identifying trends, and can often result in the identification of causative factors and possible solutions.

Documenting all information

It is essential to record everything with respect to safety issues. With an ever-increasing number of legal actions being taken against service providers it is prudent to keep accurate records.

Adhering to reporting mechanisms

Members should always adhere to the organisation's policy regarding 'lines of communication'. Misinformation or incomplete information is a major cause of failure to implement change.

Hazards and risks

A hazard is a situation with the potential to harm life, health, or property. All hazards should be documented. Table 20.1 (page 250) provides examples of hazards that are commonly found in aged-care facilities.

Major causes of hazards include:
▶ poor training and competencies;
▶ poor design and unsafe operation of equipment;
▶ stress on the job;
▶ exposure to harmful substances and processes;
▶ inadequate maintenance;
▶ lack of signage; and
▶ poor working conditions.

Once a hazard has been identified, a risk analysis should be undertaken. This involves ascertaining how frequently people are exposed to the hazard. For example, in the case of an uneven floor surface, an assessment needs to be made of how often the floor surface is traversed and by how many people.

Table 20.1 Hazards and potential harm

Hazards	Examples of potential harm
Loose floor coverings, leads across floors, spillage, wet floors, uneven surfaces	Slips, trips, falls, electrocution
Inadequate lighting	Slips, trips, falls
Faulty equipment	Injuries, electrocution
Unattended medicines, chemicals	Poisoning
Excessive noise	Dysfunctional behaviour, hearing impairment
Lack of security	Residents becoming lost or absconding
Physical restraints	Injuries (fractures, skin tears, and so on)
Smoking	Fires, burns, passive-smoking risks
Vehicle travel	Traffic accidents
Biological waste products	Infection
Extremes of temperature	Sunburn, hypothermia

Authors' creation

All risks should be minimised or eliminated. The Box below contains a list of actions (in order of priority) for risk minimisation.

Risk minimisation

The following steps (in order of priority) should be undertaken to reduce exposure to risk:
- remove, eliminate, or reduce the hazard;
- substitute or replace the hazard (for example, one chemical being replaced with another);
- redesign equipment or change process;
- enclose the hazard (for example, acoustic muffling);
- segregate from the hazard (for example, rotating members of a group);
- administrative change (for example, policies and procedures);
- provide personal protective equipment.

Adapted from WH&S 1989

Accidents and incidents

Once an accident or incident has occurred and any necessary first-aid measures have been administered, prompt investigation and analysis of the situation should be undertaken. All data should be recorded, including:

- a full description of the accident or incident;
- outcomes;
- probable cause;
- risk-assessment results;
- risk analysis;
- preventive actions; and
- 'close-out' date.

Emergency systems

All older people's services need to have written policies and procedures in place in case of an emergency situation. However, formal documentation is insufficient to ensure safety in an emergency situation, and regular (at least bi-annual) 'mock' exercises should be conducted and evaluated. Examples of emergency situations that require policies and procedures to be in place are:

> 'Formal documentation is insufficient to ensure safety in an emergency situation.'

- fire;
- building and area evacuation;
- bomb threat;
- invasion;
- impact;
- storms, cyclones, floods and other natural disasters;
- chemical spills; and
- failure of vital services (electricity, gas, water, sewerage).

Emergency policies should be formulated in conjunction with relevant local authorities (such as police, fire services, emergency services, and local municipal personnel).

Conclusion

Ensuring and maintaining a safe environment in older people's services is fundamental to the protection of older people and their living environment.

'Nurses are responsible for safety issues within their own workplaces to protect themselves and those in their care.'

Older people are highly vulnerable to hazards and risks because they are often unable to protect themselves. Older people's nurses must therefore be responsible for safety issues within their own workplaces to protect themselves and those in their care.

Chapter 21

Elder Abuse

Alex Yui-huen Kwan

Introduction

Over the past decade or so, social and economic pressures have forced Western governments to focus on policies that address the needs of the older population. The recognition of 'elder abuse' as a social issue has coincided with this focus on the aged and, in particular, on the more vulnerable sections of the aged population. In the UK, Sumner (2002) suggests that recognition of the issue is due to broadening of research into abuse of vulnerable adults in the 1970s and 1980s. The scale of abuse which was identified triggered wider debate over the last twelve years, with the establishment of networks such as the International Network for the Prevention of Elder Abuse (INPEA), and campaigning organisations such as Action on Elder Abuse, POPAN and VOICE UK.

There is no doubt that the abuse of older people occurs both in the community and in healthcare institutions. Nurses, whether based in hospitals or in the community, are in an ideal position to identify possible abuse. However, to be able to carry out this role, they need specific education, training, and guidance to heighten their awareness (Davies 1994).

The emergence of elder abuse

The term 'elder abuse' appears to have developed from the work of Baker (1975), after which it steadily gained prominence in the field of health and social welfare, and in academic social gerontology. The term refers to any harm or neglect done to an older person that is violent or abusive. The abuse can be caused by a family member, by a friend, by staff members (in group residential settings), or by anyone upon whom the older person relies for basic needs (Kosberg 1988; Ministry of Citizenship 1991; Council of Europe 1992). However, despite the consensus about the general nature of elder abuse, there remains disagreement about the details of what does and does not count as 'abuse' (Giordano & Giordano 1984; Hudson & Johnson 1987; Moore & Thompson 1987; Schlesinger & Schlesinger 1988; Hugman 1995).

There is also controversy over whether 'elder abuse' has recently increased in prevalence, whether it has been occurring for a long time but has only just come to the attention of professionals and academics (who are now more attuned to the issue, or less prejudicial towards the needs of older people), or even whether it has emerged as a product of professionals and academics creating new areas of expertise for themselves (Callahan 1988; Kosberg 1988; Leroux & Petrunik 1990; Kurrle, Sadler & Cameron 1991).

Causes

Unfortunately, the general attitude towards older people, particularly in healthcare settings, tends to be negative. This view can be held by staff members working within such units, as well as by people outside. These negative attitudes are brought about by (Davies 1994):

▶ a perceived lack of professional progression in this sector of nursing;
▶ low-level staffing and inappropriate skill mixes, which cause staff members to choose procedures of care that are incompatible with the ideal of good practice or with their codes of professional conduct;
▶ the perception that finances go to 'high-tech' areas, at the expense of care of older people; and
▶ low sponsorship potential.

Specialising in work with older people is thus often seen as a low-status branch of medicine, nursing, social work, and remedial therapy (Slevin 1991). However, there is a danger that attempts to lift the status of carers in this area might create a 'bandwagon effect' that promotes careers without helping service users (Callahan (1988).

Whatever the precise nature of the causes of elder abuse, the work of professionals in this area has definitely established the fact of violence or neglect towards older people who are dependent on others for some aspect of daily life. How- ever, the recognition of elder abuse has taken longer to become accepted

> 'The recognition of elder abuse has taken longer to become accepted as a problem.'

as a problem, compared with, say, domestic violence. This might, itself, be a result of the widespread ambivalence towards older people.

Types of abuse

Although there is no full consensus on the classification of elder abuse, the following categories have been suggested (Dolon & Hendricks 1989):

▶ *physical abuse:* slapping, pushing, hitting, restraining, bruising, burning, cutting, and so on;
▶ *psychological abuse:* insulting, blaming, ignoring, humiliating, isolating, blackmailing, swearing at, treating as a child or calling names;
▶ *material/financial abuse:* illegal or unethical exploitation of funds, property, assets, pensions, or other money; outright theft, fraud, and damage to possessions;
▶ *social/physical isolation:* abandonment or locking away in rooms;
▶ *passive neglect:* unintentional failure to fulfil care needs (for example, non-provision of food);
▶ *active neglect:* intentional failure to fulfil care needs (for example, deliberate abandonment and/or denial of food or medicine);
▶ *self-abuse/neglect:* abuse of alcohol or other drugs; inappropriate diet; failure to exercise personal care.
▶ *sexual abuse:* rape, perversion, or molestation;
▶ *violation of rights:* withholding information; domination of elderly people to force certain decisions; and
▶ *late-onset spouse abuse:* apart from domestic abuse in marriage that has been present for many years, abuse can also be triggered late in a marriage because of certain age-related factors.

Elder abuse in institutions
Staff issues
Elder abuse within residential settings is complicated and harder to define and detect than abuse within the family or community services.

Two categories of maltreatment have been identified (Fleishman & Ronen 1989):

▶ acts of omission (including passive and active neglect); and

▶ acts of commission (including physical and psychological abuse, the violation of rights and liberties, and financial and personal exploitation).

Acts of omission can refer to situations in which residents with visual or hearing difficulties do not see specialists or obtain the appropriate assistance—thereby limiting their autonomy and social activities.

Acts of commission, such as the violation of residents' rights (even to the point of physical and psychological abuse) are mainly perpetuated by nurses' aides. Such abuse includes treating older people as children, calling them names, shouting, threatening, and ignoring their requests. Given the strain under which many healthcare professionals work in institutional care, it is to be expected that exasperation and anger will occasionally erupt.

> 'Given the strain under which many healthcare professionals work in institutional care, it is to be expected that exasperation and anger will occasionally erupt.'

Resident issues

Examples of ill-treatment and abuse can also come from older people themselves. This might be a consequence of dementia or of a stroke, or it might even represent the norm for that person.

Being disabled can also be a risk factor. The experience of being dependent can provoke a violent reaction from within a disabled person—and walking sticks or wheelchairs can make very effective weapons.

Family and cultural issues

Family issues can also be a factor in elder abuse. Even if older people are residing in institutions, their relationships with their family members often remain strong and complex, and these can produce ethical and professional problems for staff members. These problems can be due to personal and family perspectives, or to particular cultural norms.

In terms of personal and family issues, many older residents resist a formal institutional system, especially when they perceive this to be punitive to their families. They might have a reluctance to 'wash dirty linen' outside the family network. Many wish to protect their children—however abusive those children might be towards them. Others might harbour guilt for raising such children.

There are also cultural issues that play a part in producing ethical and professional problems for staff. For example, in certain immigrant groups wife-beating is part of a familial-ethnic culture and is not considered abuse. Patterns of family violence can be a continuation of a 30–40-year lifestyle. In some cultural groups there is such a strong commitment to the concept of 'family' that the formal institutional system is considered to be the 'enemy.' In these circumstances, the norm is to keep things within the extended network.

> 'A strong commitment to the concept of "family" can mean that the formal institutional system is considered to be the "enemy".'

Ethical dilemmas

The above discussion of the issues involved in elder abuse brings into focus significant ethical dilemmas for staff. The issues involved—staff, personal, family, and cultural—are complex, and the dilemmas are not easily resolved. This is especially relevant in those jurisdictions in which mandatory reporting is practised (or is being promoted as policy). These include the following.

▶ Mandatory reporting of elder abuse could adversely affect resident–staff relationships––especially in the very sensitive area of family relations. The issue of confidentiality is crucial here. Should the emphasis be on treatment or should a punitive approach be used?

▶ It is often difficult to convince older people to press charges against staff members. In some cases overt abuse is difficult to establish, and older people often adjust to situations in which they perceive themselves to be powerless. If an older person makes such an 'adjustment', it can be difficult to establish that the original staff actions (which caused the 'adjustment') should still be considered as 'abuse'.

▶ Verbal and financial 'misdemeanours' are not, in most jurisdictions, formally considered to be abusive. Should such cases, if detected, be reported, or should they merely be dealt with in the framework of 'counselling'? It is sometimes difficult to differentiate between a 'misdemeanour' and outright abuse.

Detecting elder abuse

The majority of people who are admitted to hospitals and residential-care units are in a poor state of health—physically, psychologically, or socially. The majority have multiple problems. In these circumstances, signs of physical abuse and neglect are often not readily apparent, and there might be little overt evidence to raise suspicion. However, nurses should be aware of possible indicators of abuse. These are listed in the Box below.

Indicators of elder abuse

Physical abuse and neglect are often not readily apparent. However, nurses should be aware of possible signs of abuse. These include the following:

- undue anxiety or aggression displayed by an older person;
- depression, helplessness, or hopelessness;
- questions suggesting fearfulness of what is being done, or fearfulness of being left alone (such as: 'What are you going to do to me?');
- ribbons in hair, toys, and baby talk;
- cowering;
- expressions of ambivalent feelings towards family;
- excessively tired, confused, or tearful;
- marked insomnia;
- unusual interest being shown (by others) in the older person's possessions, especially money;
- necessities not being provided by carers (for example, lack of money for soap, sweets, and newspapers) despite carers' holding the pension and/or bank books; and
- the person being distressed by being 'forced' to sign unexplained legal and financial documents.

Adapted from Davies (1994)

If a resident has relatives, the best indicator that all is not well is evidence of stress in the former carer. However, most carers exhibit some signs of stress, and the role of the nurse is to attempt to measure the intensity of feeling associated with the common signals that might be expected in carers. Signs of stress in carers that should be noted by nurses are listed in the Box on page 259.

In some circumstances investigation will be necessary. Such investigations should include developing communication, building a relationship, and the exercise of negotiating, bargaining, and advocacy skills. The following preliminaries have been suggested (Kent Social Services Department 1989):

- visiting with another staff member;
- explaining the purpose of the visit;
- interviewing the dependent elder alone;

Signs of stress in carers

Signs of undue stress in carers can be an indication of elder abuse in some circumstances. Although most carers exhibit some signs of stress, nurses should be alert to the following:

- frequent requests for help (from carer or patient), including frequent requests for admission to care;
- signs of aggression, frustration, or despair—often directed towards staff members;
- obvious signs of physical or mental illness, or exhaustion;
- no visits or telephone enquiries from carers;
- non-participation in discharge planning;
- anxiety and worry, expressions of feeling isolated and lonely; evidence of low self-esteem or depression;
- indifferent relationship with patient;
- obvious alcohol or other drug dependence; and
- over-critical attitudes regarding aspects of patient care.

Adapted from Davies (1994)

◗ interviewing the caregiver separately afterwards; and
◗ arranging appropriate interpreting services if required.

Furthermore, it is appropriate to consider the manner of the interview. General good practice has shown that a conversational style, a relaxed atmosphere, remaining non-judgmental, and avoiding leading questions are all important. It is also important to *look* for clues (as well as listening), and to assess the mental capacity of the person being interviewed (Manthorpe 1994).

Moreover, time and sensitivity are particularly relevant when there are communication disorders. To compensate for some of the memory deficits and other deficits that are common in older people who suffer from dementia, it is important to optimise the environment (with good lighting, little noise, and close seating positions), to maintain eye contact and body contact, to validate the feelings behind an apparently inappropriate comment, to reorientate the person when required, to give time for responses (repeating questions when necessary), and to pay close attention to following the 'thread' of the conversation (Jones 1992).

In summary, nurses who work with abuse cases must be alert, positive, and non-threatening if they are to detect the signs of abuse and establish the needed rapport to investigate it professionally.

Designing an intervention strategy

After the detection of a suspected case of elder abuse, the most important challenge to be faced is the design and implementation of a non-threatening intervention strategy. In designing a strategy to deal with elder abuse, the following barriers should be noted (Eckley & Vilakazi 1995):

- possible lack of alternatives to family care, and an inability to escape;
- possible social taboos about invading family privacy;
- the severe emotions involved in reporting an abuser;
- victims hiding facts (due to the fear of further abuse); and
- fear of possible institutionalisation.

Having taken account of the individual factors and possible barriers operating in any given case, nurses need to work with other professionals to devise and implement a suitable intervention strategy for the protection and well-being of those in their care.

Conclusion

Nurses must continue to become more sensitive and responsive to the issue of actual and potential abuse by acknowledging that the problem does exist among elderly members of the population. They must be willing to ask difficult and sensitive questions about the appearance of bruises, fractures, or other untoward injuries in older patients, and they must be alert to the other (more subtle) signs of abuse (as discussed in this chapter).

Health care is no longer only about curing diseases. It now encompasses rehabilitation and the prevention of illness. The nurse has much to offer in the area of elder abuse, and the rewards are worth the effort made.

'The nurse has much to offer in the area of elder abuse, and the rewards are worth the effort made.'

Chapter 22

Communicating in Frustrating Situations

Jacie-Lee Whitfield

Introduction

Frustrating situations experienced by nurses can usually be directly attributed to difficulties associated with communication. Communication breakdown is one of the primary sources of stress for nurses, and communication barriers are often evident during various interactions—for example, in communication with people with dementia or with people from different cultural and linguistic backgrounds.

As the population ages and migration continues, nurses can expect older, frailer, and more culturally diverse people to enter Care Homes, and they can expect an increasing incidence of dementia among those residents. In these circumstances, it might be expected that the skilled workforce to serve such needs would similarly increase. Unfortunately, staff shortages and the employment of unregulated and undereducated staff are common in Care Homes. Such deficiencies elevate stress levels among nurses, and increase the likelihood of fatigue, injury, and job dissatisfaction (Beck et al. 1999).

262 | Chapter 22

In providing care for persons with dementia, or those from a culturally and linguistically different background, nurses can experience feelings of anger and helplessness as they attempt to manage challenging behaviour. This can lead to hasty interactions, which, in turn, infringe on the resident's rights to participate in care, make decisions, and communicate needs. In addition, nurses can feel anxious about their own safety when working with physically aggressive residents. Finally, the pressure to complete daily care tasks can mean that nurses have little opportunity to reflect on their practice, or to verbalise their concerns.

To cope with situations that cause stress and frustration, nurses should augment their repertoire of skills that have worked in the past, attempt new strategies that can de-escalate stressful situations, and take actions that will decrease their own levels of frustration. There are no 'easy fixes' or miracle solutions—because the cause of increased stress and frustration levels is directly related to the inability to cope effectively with the presenting situation. Often nurses experience a sense of failure when they are unable to manage a situation, but realistically this reaction is unreasonable. Nurses should not blame themselves when confronted with awkward and frustrating situations. They have always occurred in nursing, and they will continue to present themselves.

> 'There are no 'easy fixes' or miracle solutions.'

Frustrating situations

A list of frustrating situations in Care Homes would be endless. An isolated event is not usually frustrating—and *can* be managed. Indeed, such isolated problems are managed successfully in the course of every working day in Care Homes. It is when several situations are occurring simultaneously that stress levels soar.

Frustrating situations originate from many sources. They can be caused by residents, by the family, friends, or representatives of residents, by employees and employers, by personal issues, and by environmental factors. Some frustrating situations are shown in Table 22.1 (page 263).

Table 22.1 Frustrating situations

Resident-centred	Environment-centred	Other
Perseveration	Excessive noise	Inadequate staff/
Repetitive actions	Uncomfortable temperatures	resident ratio
and requests	Cluttered environment	Staff shortages,
Screaming, yelling	Insufficient equipment	absenteeism, sick leave
Wandering	Insufficient supplies	Organising staff
Intrusiveness	Inadequate lighting	replacements
Attempts to abscond	Lack of diversional or	Poor staff skill mix
Resistiveness	recreational activities	Inadequate knowledge
Verbal and physical	System failures	or experience
aggression		Excessive workloads
Unreasonable requests		Excessive documentary
Vexatious complaints		requirements
Difficulties with		Poor perception of
language interpretation		status, remuneration,
Declining care provision		and prestige
Risk-taking behaviours		Personal problems

Authors' creation

With regard to the list in the 'resident-centred' column of Table 22.1, it must be stressed that people with dementia act out their needs symbolically. Their behaviour is often interpreted as being deliberate in intent, but this is unfair and unreasonable. Dementia is an organic brain disorder, and is classified as a psychosis. It is therefore inappropriate to think in terms of 'deliberate intent'. However, nurses should not ignore vocal and disruptive behaviour—because every expression from a resident with dementia is an attempt to communicate (Finnema et al. 2000).

> 'It is inappropriate to think in terms of "deliberate intent".'

Frustrating situations originating from residents' family members, friends, or representatives can sometimes be rationalised by applying knowledge of the 'grief process'. These people have placed their loved one in an institution, and many of them are grieving their loss. The grieving process often involves feelings of anger, guilt, and helplessness, and these feelings are sometimes externalised in the form of unreasonable requests, complaints, and intrusiveness. Constant sharing of information, involvement in care, and genuine empathy are helpful in dissipating anxieties and defusing potentially volatile situations.

Dementia and communication

Some of the communication difficulties produced by dementia include:
- deterioration of language and memory skills;
- reiteration of words and/or sentences;
- constant retelling of stories and use of repetitive dialogue that is often rambling and littered with seemingly meaningless speech;
- lack of concentration and interest, especially when involved in communication;
- inability to process language due to poor auditory comprehension;
- failure to initiate speech;
- excessive use of speech;
- inability to find appropriate words for expression;
- decline in sensory functions (for example, eyesight, hearing, taste, smell, and touch);
- inability to recognise visual and other stimuli causing disorientation and misperception;
- limited visual field and diminished visual perspicacity;
- altered disposition, including depression and irritability;
- psychological symptoms, including delusions and hallucinations; and
- indecisiveness or limited decision-making ability.

Adapted from Done & Thomas (2001); Ward (2002)

Frustrating environmental situations are best ameliorated by continuous quality improvement, development and implementation of contingency plans (as the need arises), and effective communication throughout the structure of the organisation.

Some of the situations listed in the column entitled 'Other' in Table 22.1 are, unfortunately, all too common in the aged-care industry. Most older people's nurses are exemplary practitioners whose expertise and specialist status are not properly acknowledged within the healthcare industry. Indeed, their expertise and status are often not acknowledged by older people's nurses themselves! Contemporary older people's nursing is a dynamic specialty area that is worthy of prestige. Positive 'self-talk', assertive communication, and increased self-esteem will significantly diminish most of the frustrating situations listed under 'Other' in Table 22.1. If nurses feel good about themselves, and are professional, assertive, and confident of their value to health care, many of these issues will be resolved before frustration sets in.

Different cultural and linguistic background

People from a different linguistic and cultural background face additional difficulties in communication. In these circumstances, communication can also be hindered by:

- preferred use of a foreign language;
- limited experience and use of the English language;
- stereotyping and discrimination with respect to class, gender, ethnicity, sexuality, age, religion, and culture;
- lack of interpreters, lack of bilingual/multilingual staff, and need to rely on informal interpreters (with a conflict of interest being possible);
- foreign cultural traditions and rules; and
- use of degrading language that belittles residents.

Adapted from Queensland Health (1998)

Communication difficulties

Dementia

Older people's nurses are fully cognisant of the fact that dementia can impede a person's ability to communicate. The Box on page 264 lists some of the communication difficulties produced by dementia.

Culture and language

Nurses are also cognisant that communication can also be hindered if residents are from different cultures or if their primary language is foreign to the language in common use. The Box above provides a list of some of the communication problems experienced by these people.

Dealing with frustrating situations

Being fully aware of these communication barriers is the foundation upon which nurses and carers can base their action plan to prevent, defuse, or resolve frustrating situations. All action plans should emerge from a comprehensive knowledge of the resident's history, any specific cultural and ethnic needs, and the person's preferences and idiosyncrasies.

Some actions to augment the nurses' professional repertoire of coping mechanisms include:

- utilising a specific theoretical model of gerontic care;
- activity programs;

266 | Chapter 22
NURSING OLDER PEOPLE

- validating feelings;
- reminiscence;
- emotion centred care;
- simulated presence therapy (SPT); and
- stress-management techniques.

Each of these is discussed below.

Utilising a specific theoretical model

Many theoretical models of older people's nursing can be found within the literature. Some models advocate minimal stimulation whereas others, on the other end of the continuum, suggest intensive stimulation. No matter which model is selected, it should be chosen with the individual's needs and ethnicity in mind. What works for one person will not necessarily work for another. Some models will need to be adjusted or modified to suit both the resident and the Care Home. The chosen model should be effective in reducing the occurrence of dysfunctional behaviours.

Activity programs

Institutionalisation contributes to a number of negative outcomes. Such negative outcomes include boredom, depression, isolation, withdrawal, self-absorption, and, sometimes, suicidal ideation. These are often manifested as dysfunctional behaviour.

'Institutionalisation . . . is often manifested as dysfunctional behaviour.'

It is vitally important that activity programs are implemented within Care Homes. The programs should offer alternatives—with more than one activity at a time being available. The heterogeneous nature of the group means that one activity will not suit all. Because older people require less sleep than do younger adults, it is also important that activities should be offered throughout the day. Residents should be encouraged to attend, but should certainly not be forced or coerced. Socialisation with peers will markedly reduce negative outcomes and dysfunctional behaviour.

As John F. Kennedy stated (Pinkney & Whiter (1997):

> There are risks and costs to a program of action. But they are far less than the long-range risks and costs of comfortable inaction.

Validating feelings

The feelings of any person are only rarely expressed overtly or verbally. Feelings are generally expressed symbolically and couched in complex speech that presents the recipient, at the best of times, with a virtual conundrum to unravel. The analysis of the enigma is further compounded when a resident has dementia. Validating feelings of a person with dementia can best be achieved by attempting to confirm feelings using the same modality as the person using to express his or her perception of reality. These modalities include body language, paralanguage, and visual, auditory and kinaesthetic communicative styles (Finnema et al. 2000).

Although the term 'body language' is in common usage, the term 'paralanguage' is less common and less well understood. 'Paralanguage' includes pitch, tone, and volume of speech. The use of touch, light, sound, music, and colours will often authenticate a person's feelings and allay any negativity associated with his or her expressed experience. Any extraneous noises should be reduced because persons with dementia have a reduced ability to filter out such 'interference' (Ward 2002). Mirroring the actions of the resident without imitating his or her anger or threats will assist in validating the person's feelings and reduce future repetition of behaviours that express anxiety, guilt, or fear (Feil 1993).

> 'Mirroring the actions of the resident without imitating his or her anger will assist in validating the person's feelings.'

The preferred communicative style of a person can be ascertained by noting the following (Meier 2002).

▶ A 'visual' person uses words to recall and describe pictures stored in the memory. Visual communicators use 'describing words', such as 'see', 'look', 'appear', 'imagine', and 'picture'. These people attempt to view the picture in their minds, willing the eyes upwards, and often blinking to clarify images.

▶ An 'auditory' person engages frequently in dialogue and converses internally using words such as 'hear', 'listen', and 'sound'. In communication, auditory people divert the eyes to the side, often repeating questions or statements.

▶ A 'kinaesthetic' person is concerned with feeling and will sometimes rely on intuition in communication. These people might recall the taste and smell of situations when reminiscing, and use words such as 'touch', 'feel', and 'impression'.

Using the preferred communicative style of a person in any interaction enhances the interchange of ideas, thoughts, and feelings.

Reminiscence

'Reminiscing usually involves a relationship between a storyteller and one or more listeners' (Forster 2003). By imparting memories the associated emotions are shared. Reminiscence is particularly useful when attempting to communicate with people with dementia—because an ability to feel emotional about the past is usually retained. Reminiscence therapy is intended to support the recollection of memories in a non-threatening manner.

Reminiscence can be used in a group activity to encourage resident socialisation or in a one-on-one approach to stimulate interest and improve disposition. For severely impaired residents, the use of photographs, personal objects, and music can be more suitable than vocalisation (Finnema et al. 2000). Helga's story (Box, below) illustrates the effectiveness of reminiscence.

Helga

Helga, an 82-year-old German woman, had moved to England twenty years ago. She had been admitted to a nursing home when she was 76 years old with a diagnosis of end-stage dementia.

Helga was bed-fast and spent her time kicking the bedclothes and calling out in German. All nursing interventions to reduce her obvious anxiety were unsuccessful.

One day, Helga's daughter brought in a tape recording of German lullabies and some of Helga's favourite songs from her courting days. When the tape was played, Helga smiled, stopped kicking, listened to the music, and attempted to hum the tunes.

Reminiscence had been remarkably successful in alleviating anxiety when all other interventions had been ineffective.

Emotion-centred care

To facilitate the reduction of frustrating situations and enhance interaction with residents, nurses might wish to utilise the techniques of emotion-centred care (Finnema et al. 2000). Emotion-centred care includes approaches that focus on the emotional capabilities of residents—such as validating feelings, reminiscence, laughter therapy, touch, music, movement therapy, and simulated presence therapy. Care must be taken in these approaches to ensure that the unique needs of people with dementia are addressed.

Emotion-centred care relies upon an environment that nurtures unconditional acceptance of each individual and supports the candid expression of feelings. An empathic attitude is essential when employing emotion-centred care, and each approach can be developed to benefit the care recipient and the nurse so that all interactions are enjoyable.

Emotion-centred care is a positive approach to reducing dysfunctional behaviour in residents with dementia because an intact memory is not required to laugh and have fun.

'An intact memory is not required to laugh and have fun.'

Simulated presence therapy

Simulated presence therapy (SPT) aims to simulate the presence of a trusted friend or relative known to the resident before admission. This person symbolises a fundamental source of security and stability for the resident. Therapy involves the recreation of significant experiences that stimulate positive behaviour and feelings.

An example of SPT is 'video-respite'—whereby video footage of autobiographical stories and memories is played to reduce aggression, wandering, repetitive questioning, and argumentative behaviour in residents (Finnema et al. 2000). Video respite is particularly useful in situations in which residents display repeated concern for relatives, friends, lost items, or objects presumed stolen.

Other examples of STP include 'audio letters' and recorded reminiscence sessions. These can provide comfort to residents in times of anxiety and distress. Norma's story (Box, below) illustrates the effectiveness of SPT.

Norma

Norma, a 76-year-old woman, had been admitted to a nursing home with a diagnosis of Alzheimer's dementia ten years previously. When her memory markedly deteriorated and she started to lose her belongings, her son took some family heirlooms home. Following the removal of her belongings, Norma spent all of her days searching for the objects and repeatedly asking staff where her items were.

A videotape recording was made of the son at home, explaining that he had the objects and showing Norma where they were.

Whenever Norma enquired about her 'lost' belongings, nurses played the tape for her, and this reduced her immediate anxiety. After two weeks her searching activities and continual questions noticeably decreased.

Nurses' self-care

It is important that nurses and carers look after themselves. To decrease stress in frustrating situations, laughter is often a good antidote. Having the ability to laugh at adverse situations relieves tension, facilitates work effectiveness, promotes creativity, assists in the retention of information, increases intellectual performance, and puts problems into perspective.

Other aspects of self-care and stress management include:

- using anger-management techniques, asserting personal power, positive self-talk, and so on;
- using problem-solving techniques;
- seeking social support (family, friends, and colleagues);
- participating in counselling programs;
- exercising (partaking of at least 20 minutes of exercise daily);
- relaxing (mentally and physically);
- participating in committees, meetings, and work-improvement programs;
- participating in educational activities;
- setting realistic, short-term, medium-term, and long-term goals;
- giving and receiving praise for achievements;
- acting immediately to prevent tension as soon as internal feelings of stress are noted;
- processing traumatic information in 'tolerable doses' to prevent being overwhelmed with panic; and
- practising stress-management techniques (such as tai-chi, yoga, self-hypnotic induction, visualisation, positive affirmations, neuro-linguistic programming, and meditation.

Conclusion

Experiencing frustration and stress can result in nurses and carers being depressed or feeling angry, anxious, and guilty. Although negative in connotation, these feelings can be responded to in a healthy manner—which will assist in the prevention of recurring frustration, abuse, burnout, depression, and discontentment (Beck et al. 1999).

References

Chapter 1 Aged Care Nursing

Care Standards Act 2000, The Stationery Office, London.

Cluning, T. (ed.) 2001, *Ageing at Home—Practical Approaches to Community Care*, Ausmed Publications, Melbourne.

Eliopoulos, C. 1987, *Gerontological Nursing*, 2nd edn, J.B. Lippincott Company, Philadelphia.

Engel, G.L. 1977, 'The Need for a New Medical Model: A Challenge for Biomedicine', *Science*, 196, pp 129–36.

Gray, L., Woodward, M., Scholes R., Busby W. & Fonda D. 2000, *Geriatric Medicine—A Pocket Guide for Doctors, Nurses, Other Health Professionals and Students*, 2nd edn, Ausmed Publications, Melbourne.

Neugarten, B.L. 1970, 'Dynamics of transition of middle age to old age adaption and the life cycle', *Journal of Geriatric Psychiatry*, 4, pp 71–87.

Secretary of State for Health 2001, National Minimum Standards for Older People. The Stationery Office, London.

Chapter 2 Nursing Assessments

Cluning, T. (ed.) 2001, *Ageing at Home—Practical Approaches to Community Care*, Ausmed Publications, Melbourne.

Department of Health and Aged Care 1999, *Documentation and Accountability Manual*, Commonwealth of Australia, Canberra.

Engel, G.L. 1977, 'The Need for a New Medical Model: A Challenge for Biomedicine', *Science*, 196, pp 129–36.

Holmes, H.N. (ed.) 1997, *Mastering Geriatric Care*, Springhouse Corporation, Springhouse, USA.

Holmes, H.N. (ed.) 1999, *Handbook of Geriatric Nursing Care*, Springhouse Corporation, Springhouse, USA.

Chapter 3 Skin and Oral Hygiene

Agency for Health Care Policy and Research 1992, Publication No. 92-0047, May 1992, 'Pressure Ulcers in Adults: Prediction and Prevention', Clinical Practice Guidelines, Number 3, US Department of Health and Human Services, Public Health Service.

AHCPR, *see* Agency for Health Care Policy and Research.

Aronowitz, S.A. 1997, 'Oral care and its role in wound, ostomy-continence nursing', *Journal of Wound Ostomy-Continence Nursing*, 24: 2, 79–84.

Ayliffe, G.A., Collins, B.J. & Taylor, L.J. 1985, *Hospital Acquired Infection, Principle and Prevention*, 2nd edn, Wright Publishing, London.

Beck, S. & Yasko, J. 1993, *Guidelines for Oral Care*, 2nd edn, Sage, Crystal Lake, USA.

Beck, S. & Yasko, J. 2001, 'Oral Care. The Inside Story', Nursing Institute, May 2001, <www.sageproducts.com/education>.

Frantz, R.A. & Kinney, C.N. 1986, 'Variables Associated with Skin Dryness in the Elderly', *Nursing Research*, 35: 98–100.

Kabara, J.J. & Brady, M.G. 1984, 'Contamination of Bar Soaps Under 'in-use' Conditions', *Journal of Environmental Pathology, Toxicology and Oncology*, 5: 1–14.

Mason, S.R. 1997, 'Type of Soap and the Incidence of Skin Tears among Residents of a Long-Term Care Facility', *Ostomy Wound Management*, Sept, 43(8): 26–30.

McGough-Csarny J. & Kopac, C.A. 1998, 'Skin Tears in Institutionalized Elderly: an Epidemiological Study', *Ostomy/Wound Management*, 44(3A): 14S–25S.

Nam, K. & Gracey, D.R. 1972, 'Pulmonary talcosis from cosmetic powder', *Journal of American Medical Association*, July, vol. 221: 492–3.

Nix, D. 2000, 'Factors to consider when selecting skin cleansing products', *Journal of Wound, Ostomy and Continence Nursing*, 27: 260–8.

Passos, J. & Brand, L. 1966, 'Effects of Agents Used for Oral Hygiene', *Nursing Research*, 15: 196–202.

Chapter 4 Pressure Ulcers and Leg Ulcers

Australian Wound Management Association 2001, *Clinical Practice Guidelines for the Prediction and Prevention of Pressure Ulcers*, Cambridge Publishing, West Leederville, Australia.

AWMA, *see* Australian Wound Management Association.

Banks, V. 1998, 'Pressure Sore Risk Assessment', *Journal of Wound Care*, 7(2): 91–2.

Braden, B. & Bergstrom, N. 1987, 'A conceptual scheme for the study of the etiology of pressure sores, *Rehabilitation Nursing*, 12(1): 8–16.

Bryant, R.A. (ed.) 1992, *Acute and Chronic Wounds: Nursing Management*, Mosby Year Book, St Louis, Missouri, USA.

Bryant, R.A., Shannon, M.L., Pieper, B., Braden, B.J. & Morris, D.J. 1992, 'Pressure Ulcers', in Bryant 1992, op. cit., pp 105–52.

Carville, K. 2001, *Wound Care Manual*, Silver Chain Foundation, Osborne Park, Western Australia.

Cullum, N. & Roe, B. 1998, *Leg Ulcers: Nursing Management—A research based guide*, Bailliére Tindall, London, England.

Cullum, N., Fletcher, A.W., Nelson, E.A. & Sheldon, T.A. 1998, 'Compression bandages and stockings in the treatment of venous leg ulcers', Cochrane Review, *The Cochrane Library*, Issue 4.

Dealey, C. 1994, *The Care of Wounds*, Blackwell Scientific Publications, Oxford, UK.

Doughty, D.B. 1992, 'Principles of Wound Healing and Wound Management', in Bryant 1992, op. cit., pp 31–61.

Falanga, V. 2001, *Science of Wound Management: Wound Bed Preparation*, Smith & Nephew, Hull, UK.

Fergusson, J.A.E. & MacLellan, D.G. 1997, 'Wound Management in Older People', *The Australian Journal of Hospital Pharmacy*, 27(6).

Fletcher, A., Cullum, N. & Sheldon, T.A. 1997, 'A Systematic Review of Compression Treatment for Venous Leg Ulcers', *British Medical Journal*, (315)7108: 576–80.

Holt, D.R., Kirk, S.J., Regan, M.C., Hurson, M., Lindblad, W.J. & Barbul, A. 1992, 'Effect of Age on Wound Healing in Healthy Human Beings', *Surgery*, 112(2).

Hopkins, A. Gooch, S. & Danks, F. 1998, 'A programme for pressure sore prevention and management', *Journal of Wound Care*, 7(1): 37–40.

JBI, *see* Joanna Briggs Institute.

Joanna Briggs Institute 1997, 'Pressure Sores—Part 1: Prevention of Pressure-Related Damage', *Best Practice*, 1(1), Joanna Briggs Institute, Adelaide, Australia.

MacLellan, D.G. & Rice, J. 1995, 'Modern Wound Dressings in Acute Trauma', *Veterans Health Care*, March.

Maklebust, J. & Sieggreen, M. 2001, *Pressure Ulcers: Guidelines for Prevention and Management*, Springhouse Corporation, Pennsylvania, USA.

McLeod, A.G. 1997, 'Principles of Alternating Pressure Surfaces', *Advances in Wound Care*, 10(7): 30–6.

Morison, M., Moffatt, C., Bridel-Nixon, J. & Bale, S. 1997, *Nursing Management of Chronic Wounds*, Mosby, London, UK.

Nelson, E.A. 1996, 'Compression Bandaging in the Treatment of Venous Leg Ulcers', *Journal of Wound Care*, 5(9): 417–18.

Newman, B. & Lim, F.P. 2001, 'An Evidence Based Approach to a Perennial Problem: Pressure Ulcers', *Contemporary Nurse*, 10(1–2): 102–9.

Norton, D. 1989, 'Calculating the Risk: Reflections on the Norton Scale', *Decubitus*, 2(3): 24–31.

Pudner, R. 1997, 'Choosing an Appropriate Wound Dressing', *Journal of Community Nursing*, 11(9).

Scully, C. 1999, 'In on a Limb', *Nursing Times*, 95(27): 59–65.

Sibbald, R.G., Browne, A.C., Coutts, P. & Queen, D. 2001, 'Screening Evaluation of an Ionized Nanocrystalline Silver Dressing in Chronic Wound Care', *Ostomy Wound Management*, 47(10).

Smith, D. 2002, 'The management of mixed arterial ulcers', *Woundcare Network*, Issue 8, July.

Sundberg, J. & Meller, R. 1997, 'A Retrospective Review of the Use of Cadexomer Iodine in the Treatment of Chronic Wounds', *Wounds: A Compendium of Clinical Research and Practice*, 9(3).

Thomas, S. 1996, 'High-compression Bandages', *Journal of Wound Care*, 5(1): 40–3.
Thursby, P.F. 1993, 'Leg Ulcers: Differential Diagnosis and Management in the Elderly', *Modern Medicines of Australia*, December, 45–9.
Waterlow, J, 1985, 'A Risk-assessment Card', *Nursing Times*, 81(48): 24–7.
Vowden, K. 1998, 'Lipodermatosclerosis and Atrophie Blanche', *Journal of Wound Care*, 7(9), 441–3.

Chapter 5 Foot Care

Crawford, V.L.S., Ashford, R.L., McPeake, B. & Stout, R.W. 1995, 'Conservative Podiatric Medicine and Disability in Elderly People', *Journal of the American Podiatric Medical Association*, 85(5): 255–59.
Ebrahim, S.B.J., Sainsbury, R. & Watson, S. 1981, 'Foot Problems of the Elderly: A Hospital Survey', *British Medical Journal*, 283: 949–50.
Evans, E. & Sigurgeirsson, B. 1999, 'Double Blind, Randomised Study of Continuous Terbinafine Compared with Intermittent Itraconazole in Treatment of Toenail Onychomycosis', The LION Study Group, *British Medical Journal*, 318: 1031–5.
Flores-Rivera, A. 1998, 'Risk factors for Amputation in Diabetic Patients: A Case-Control Study', *Archives of Medical Research*, 29: 179–84.
Frey, C. 2000, 'Foot Health and Shoewear for Women', *Clinical Orthopaedics and Related Research*, 372: 32–44.
Frey, C.C., Thompson, F., Smith, J., Sanders, M. & Horstman, H. 1993, 'American Orthopedic Foot and Ankle Society Women's Shoe Survey', *Foot and Ankle*, 14(2): 78–81.
Gorecki, G. 1978, 'Shoe related Foot Problems and Public Health', *Journal of the American Podiatry Association*, 4: 242–7.
Greenberg, L. 1994, 'Foot Care Data from Two Recent Nationwide Surveys—A Comparative Analysis', *Journal of the American Podiatric Medical Association*, 84(7): 365–70.
Hart, R., Bell-Syer, S., Crawford, F., Torgerson, D., Young, P. & Russell, I. 1999, 'Systematic Review of Topical Treatments for Fungal Infections of the Skin and Nails of the Feet', *British Medical Journal*, 319: 79–82.
Hourihan, F., Cumming, R.G., Tavener-Smith, K.M. & Davidson, I. 1997, 'Footwear and Hip Fracture-related Falls in the Elderly', *Australasian Journal on Ageing*, 19: 91–3.
Hung, L., Ho, Y., Leung, P. 1985, 'Survey of Foot Deformities among 166 Geriatric Inpatients', *Foot and Ankle*, 5(4): 156–64.
Love, C. 1995 'Nursing or chiropody? Nurses' attitudes to toenail trimming', *Professional Nurse*, 10: 241–4.
Menz, H.B. & Lord, S.R. 2001, 'The Contribution of Foot Problems to Mobility Impairment and Falls in Community-Dwelling Older People', *Journal of the American Geriatrics Society*, 49: 1651–6.
Muehlman, C. & Rahimi, F. 1990, 'Aging Integumentary System. Podiatric Review', *Journal of the American Podiatric Medical Association*, 80: 577–82.
Munro, B.J. & Steele, J.R. 1998, 'Foot-Care Awareness—A Survey of Persons Aged 65 Years and Older', *Journal of the American Podiatric Medical Association*, 88(5): 242–8.
Murray, H., Young, M., Hollis, S. & Boulton, A. 1996 'The Association between Callus Formation, High Pressures and Neuropathy in Diabetic Foot Ulceration', *Diabetic Medicine*, 13: 979–82.
Pierson, M. 1991, 'Nurses' Knowledge and Perceptions Related to Foot Care for Older Persons', *Journal of Nursing Education*, 30: 57–62.
Rounding, C. & Hulm, S. 2000, 'Surgical Treatments for Ingrowing Toenails', *Cochrane Database of Systematic Reviews*, 2: CD001541.
Seale, K. 1995, 'Women and their Shoes: Unrealistic Expectations?', *Instructional Course Lectures*, 44: 379–84.
Smith, R., Katchis, S. & Ayson, L. 2000, 'Outcomes in Hallux Rigidus Patients Treated Nonoperatively: A Long-Term Follow-Up Study', *Foot and Ankle International*, 21: 906–13.
Torkki, M., Malmivaara, A., Seitsalo, S., Hoikka, V., Laippala, P. & Paavolainen, P. 2001, 'Surgery vs Orthosis vs Watchful Waiting for Hallux Valgus: A Randomized Controlled Trial', *Journal of the American Medical Association*, 285: 2474–80.
Williamson, J., Stokoe, I. & Gray, S. 1964, 'Old People at Home—Their Unreported Needs', *Lancet*, i: 1117–20.

Chapter 6 Nutrition

Pearson, A., FitzGerald, M. & Nay, R. 2003, 'Mealtimes in Nursing Homes', *Journal of Gerontological Nursing*, June, 41–7.

NHMRC, *see* National Health and Medical Research Council.
National Health and Medical Research Council 1999, *Dietary Guidelines for Older Australians*, Commonwealth of Australia, Ausinfo, Canberra.

Chapter 8 Incontinence

Abrams, P. et al. (40 co-authors) 2002, 'Evaluation and Treatment of Urinary Incontinence, Pelvic Organ Prolapse and Faecal Incontinence, *2nd International Consultation on Incontinence*, ICUD, WHO, ICS, pp 1079–117.

AHCPR, *see* Agency for Health Care Policy and Research.

Agency for Health Care Policy and Research (AHCPR) 1996, *Clinical Practice Guideline Number 2, 1996 Update: Urinary Incontinence in Adults: Acute and Chronic Management*, AHCPR, Public Health Service, US Department of Health and Human Services, Rockville, USA.

Button, D., Roe, B., Webb, C., Frith, T., Colin-Thome, D. & Gardner, L. 1998, *Consensus Guidelines, Continence Promotion and Management by the Primary Health Care Team*, Whurr, London.

Campbell, A., Reinken, J. & McCosh 1985, 'Incontinence in the Elderly: Prevalence and Prognosis', *Age and Ageing*, 14(2): 65–70.

Hunskaar, S., Arnold, E.P., Burgio, K., Diokno, A.C., Herzog, A.R. & Mallett, V.T. 1999, 'Epidemiology and Natural History of Urinary Incontinence', in Abrams, P., Khoury, S. & Wein, A. (eds), pp 197–226, *Incontinence*, Health Publication Ltd, UK.

Jilek, R. 1993, 'Elderly Toileting: Is Two-hourly Two Often?', *Nursing Standard*, 7(47), 25–6.

Lawler, J. 1991, *Behind the Screens: Nursing, Somology, and the Problem of the Body*, Churchill Livingstone: Melbourne.

Mohide, E.A. 1992, 'The Prevalence of Urinary Incontinence', in Roe, B.H. (ed.), pp 3–19, *Clinical Nursing Practice: The Promotion and Management of Continence*, Prentice Hall, London.

Norton, C. 1996, 2nd edn, *Nursing for Continence*, Beaconsfield, UK.

Norton, C. 1997, 'Faecal Incontinence in Adults 2: Treatment and Management', *British Journal of Nursing*, 6(1): 23–6.

Norton, C., Christiansen, J., Butler, U., Harari, D., Nelson, J., Permberton, K., Rovnor, E. & Sultan, A. 2002, 'Anal Incontinence', in *2nd International Consultation on Incontinence*, ICUD, WHO, ICS.

Ouslander, J.G. & Schnelle, J.F. 1995, 'Incontinence in the Nursing Home', *Annals of Internal Medicine*, 122(6): 438–49.

Ouslander, J.G., Maloney,C., Grasela, T.H., Rogers, L. & Walawander, C.A. 2001, 'Implementation of a Nursing Home Urinary Incontinence Management Program with and without Tolterodine', *Journal of the American Medical Directors Association*, 2: 207–14.

Roberts, R., Jacobsen, S., Rhodes, T., Reilly, W., Girman, C., Talley, N. & Lieber, M. 1999, 'Urinary Incontinence in a Community-based Cohort: Prevalence and Healthcare-Seeking', *Journal of the American Geriatric Society*, 46(4): 467–72.

Robinson, J.P. 2000, 'Managing Urinary Incontinence in the Nursing Home: Residents' Perspectives', *Journal of Advanced Nursing*, 31(1): 68–77.

Thom, D.H., Haan, M.N. & Van den Eeden, S.K. 1997, 'Medially Recognized Urinary Incontinence and Risks of Hospitalization, Nursing Home Admission and Mortality', *Age and Ageing*, 26: 367–74.

Yu, L.C., Johnson, K., Kaltreider, D.L., Hu, T., Brannon, D. & Ory, M. 1991, 'Urinary Incontinence: Nursing Home Staff Reaction toward Residents', *Journal of Gerontological Nursing*, 17(11).

Chapter 9 Falls

Butler, M., Norton, R., Lee-Joe, T., Cheng, A. & Campbell, J. 1996, 'The Risks of Hip Fracture in Older People from Private Homes and Institutions', *Age and Ageing*, 25: 381–5.

Davis, D. & Thomson, M. 1996, 'Implications for Undergraduate and Graduate Education Derived from Quantitative Research in Continuing Medical Education: Lessons Learned from an Automobile', *Journal of Continuing Education in the Health Professions*, 16(3): 159–66.

Hill, K., Smith, R., Murray, K., Sims, J., Gough, J., Darzins, P., Vrantsidis, F. & Clark, R. 2000, 'An Analysis of Research on Preventing Falls and Falls Injury in Older People: Community, Residential and Hospital Settings', report by the National Ageing Research Institute to the Commonwealth Department of Health and Aged Care, Canberra.

Hill, K., Vrantsidis, F., Lindeman, M., Schwarz, J., Pearce, J., McGann, A., Jessup, R., Smith, R., Barrett, C., Kronberg, M., Malkin, S. & Bryant, C. 2002, 'Preventing Adverse Events in Sub-acute Care: Changing Practice to Prevent Falls', report by the National Ageing Research Institute for the Department of Human Services (Victoria).

Lieu, P., Ismail, N., Choo, P., Kwek, P., Heng, L., Govindaraju, K. 1997, 'Prevention of Falls in a Geriatric Ward', *Annals of the Academy of Medicine*, 26(3): 266–70.

Lindeman, M., Gough, J., Smith, R., Black, K., Bryce, A., Gilsenan, B., Hill, K. & Stewart, A. 2000, 'Facilitating Change in Aged Care Residential Settings through Action Research: The Well for Life Project', paper presented at the World Congress: 5th on Action Learning, Action Research and Process Management, and 9th on Participatory Action Research, Ballarat, Victoria.

Lindeman, M., Smith, R., Vrantsidis, F. & Gough, J. 2002, 'Action Research in Aged Care. A Model for Practice Change and Development', *Geriaction*, 20(1), 10–14.

Lipsitz, L., Jonsson, P., Kelley, M. & Koestner, J. 1991, 'Causes and Correlates of Recurrent Falls in Ambulatory Frail Elderly', *Journal of Gerontology*, 46: 114–22.

Neufeld, R., Libow, L., Foley, W., Dunbar, J., Cohen, C. & Breuer, B. 1999, 'Restraint Reduction Reduces Serious Injuries among Nursing Home Residents', *Journal of the American Geriatrics Society*, 47: 1202–7.

Peninsula Health Care Network (Falls Prevention Service) 1999, *The FRAT Pack*, Peninsula Health Care Network, Mt Eliza, Victoria, Australia.

Ray, W., Taylor, J., Meador, K., Thapa, P., Brown, A., Kalihara, H., Davis, C., Gideon, P. & Griffin, M. 1997, 'A Randomised Trial of a Consultation Service to Reduce Falls in Nursing Homes', *Journal of American Medical Association*, 278(7): 557–62.

Redman, S., Boyle, F., Zorbas, H., Luxford, K., Hall, J., Gillet, D. & Andrews, K. 1999, 'Structural Change to Support Clinical Guideline Implementation: The Hospital Quality Improvement Kit Program', background papers for NHMRC's Evidence-based Clinical Practice Research Program Workshop, December 1999.

Shanley, C. 1998, *Putting Your Best Foot Forward*, Centre for Education and Research on Ageing, Concord Hospital, Concord, NSW, Report for the Commonwealth Department of Health and Aged Care.

Taylor, J. & Morris M. 1999, 'Education, Staff Knowledge and Falling in Hostel Residents', *Physiotherapy Singapore*, 2(4): 128–34.

Thapa, P., Brockman, K., Gideon, P., Fought, R. & Ray, W. 1996, 'Injurious Falls in Non-Ambulatory Nursing Home Residents: A Comparative Study of Circumstances, Incidence, and Risk Factors', *Journal of the American Geriatrics Society*, 44: 273–8.

Tinetti, M. 1987, 'Factors Associated with Serious Injury During Falls by Ambulatory Nursing Home Residents', *Journal of the American Geriatrics Society*, 35: 644–8.

van Leeuwen, M., Bennett, L., West, S., Wiles, V. & Grasso, J. 2001, 'Patient Falls from Bed and the Role of Bedrails in the Acute Care Setting', *Australian Journal of Advanced Nursing*, Dec. 19(2): 8–13.

Chapter 10 Manual Handling and Mobility

Burgess-Limerick, R. 2003, 'Squat, Stoop or Something in Between', *International Journal of Industrial Ergonomic*, 31: 143–8.

Garg, A., Owen, B., Beller, D. & Banaag, J. 1991, 'A Biomechanical and Ergonomic Evaluation of Patient Transferring Tasks: Bed to Wheelchair and Wheelchair to Bed', *Ergonomics*, 34: 289–312.

Hauer, K., Rost, B., Rutschle, K., Opitz, H., Specht, N., Bartsch, P., Oster, P. & Schlierf, G. 2001, 'Exercise Training for Rehabilitation and Secondary Prevention of Falls in Geriatric Patients with a History of Injurious Falls', *Journal of American Geriatric Society*, 2001 Jan, 49(1): 10–20.

Manual Handling Operations Regulations 1992, Statutory Instrument 1992 No 2793. The Stationery Office, London.

National Back Exchange 2001, *Manual Handling Training Guidelines* produced by a working party, chaired by Pat Alexander. <www.nationalbackexchange.org.uk>

National Back Pain Association & Royal College of Nursing 1998, *The Guide to the Handling of Patients: Introducing a Safer Handling Policy*, 4th edn, National Back Pain Association, UK.

NBPA, *see* National Back Pain Association.

NMCS 2001, See Secretary of State for Health (2001).

RCN, *see* Royal College of Nursing.

Royal College of Nursing, 1996, *Introducing a Safer Manual Handling Policy*, rev. 1996, Royal College of Nursing, UK.

Secretary of State for Health (2001) ibid.

Varcin-Coad, L. 1999, 'A Short Course in the Manual Handling of People Utilising Free-Style Lifting Techniques—Preliminary Evaluation', paper presented at 3rd National Conference on Injury Prevention and Control, Brisbane, Australia, May, 1999.

Varcin-Coad, L. 2003, *Learners Notes and Facilitator Package: LMC001 Manual Handling for Carers of People*, 4th edn, private publication, <www.manualhandling.com.au>.

Varcin-Coad, L. & Barrett, R. 1998, 'Repositioning a Slumped Patient in a Wheelchair: A Biomechanical Analysis of Three Transfer Techniques', *American Association of Occupational Health Nurses*, 46, 11, 530–6.

Varcin-Coad, L. & Stewart, M. 1999, 'Innovative Strategies for Developing Competency-based Manual Handling Training in the Health Industry', paper presented at 'Moving in on Occupational Injury', Cairns, Australia, May 1999.

Videman, T., Rauhala, H., Asp, S., Lindstrom, K., Cedercreutz, G., Kamppi, M., Tola, S. & Troup, J.D.G. 1989, 'Patient Handling Skill, Back Injuries and Back Pain: An Intervention Study', *Spine*, 14 (2), 148–56.

Yassi, A., Cooper, J.E., Tate, R.B., Gerlach, S., Muir, M., Trottier, J. & Massy, K. 2001 'A Randomised Controlled Trial to Prevent Patient Lift and Transfer Injuries of Health Care Workers', *Spine*, 26, 16: 1739–46.

Worksafe Australia 1994, *Improving Occupational Health and Safety in the Australian Health Industry— Hospital and Nursing Homes*, Steering Committee for the National OHS Strategy in the Health Industry Project.

Chapter 11 Wandering

Algase, D.L., Beck, C., Kolanowski, A., Whall, A., Berent, S., Richards, K. & Beattie, E. 1996, 'Need-driven Dementia-compromised Behavior: An Alternative View of Disruptive Behavior', *American Journal of Alzheimer's Disease*, November/December, 10–19.

Algase, D.L., Kupferschmid, B., Beel-Bates, C.A. & Beattie, E.R. 1997, 'Estimates of Stability of Daily Wandering Behavior among Cognitively Impaired Long-term Care Residents', *Nursing Research*, 46, 172–8.

Algase, D.L. 1999a, 'Wandering: A Dementia-Compromised Behavior', *Journal of Gerontological Nursing*, 25 (9), 10–16.

Algase, D.L. 1999b, 'Wandering in Dementia: State of the Science', in J.J. Fitzpatrick (ed.), 'Annual Review of Nursing Research', Springer, New York.

Algase, D.L., Beattie, E.R.A., Bogue, E. & Yao, L. 2001, 'The Algase Wandering Scale: Initial Psychometrics of a New Caregiver Reporting Tool', *American Journal of Alzheimer's Disease and Other Dementias*, 16(3), 141–52.

Algase, D.L. & Beattie, E.R.A 2002, 'Unpublished data from Wandering: Cognition & Environment', 1RO1NR04569, funded by National Institute of Aging, National Institutes of Health, Rockville, MD.

Burns, A., Jacoby, R. & Levy, R. 1990, 'Psychiatric Phenomena in Alzheimer's Disease. IV: Disorders of Behavior, *British Journal of Psychiatry*, 157, 86–94.

Cohen-Mansfield, J., Marx, M. & Rosenthal, A. 1989, 'A Description of Agitation in a Nursing Home', *Journal of Gerontology*, 44 (3), M77–84.

Cooper, J.K., Mungas, D. & Weiler, P.G. 1990, 'Relation of Cognitive Status and Abnormal Behaviors in Alzheimer's Disease', *Journal of the American Geriatrics Society*, 38, 867–70.

Cooper, J.K. & Mungas, D. 1993, 'Risk Factor and Behavioral Differences between Vascular and Alzheimer's Dementias: The Pathway to End-Stage Disease', *Journal of Geriatric Psychiatry & Neurology*, 6 (1), 29–33.

Costa, P.T. & McCrae, R.R. 1988, 'Personality in Adulthood: A Six-Year Longitudinal Study of Self Reports and Spouse Ratings on the NEO Personality Inventory', *Journal of Personality and Social Psychology*, 55, 258–65.

Costa, P.T. & McCrae, R.R. 1992, *Revised NEO Personality Inventory and NEO Five-Factor Inventory: Professional Manual*, Psychological Assessment Resources Inc., Odessa, USA.

Feldt, K. 2000, 'Checklist of Non-verbal Pain Indicators', *Pain Management Nursing*, 1 (1), 13–21.

Folstein, M.F., Folstein, S.E. & McHugh, P.R. 1975, 'Mini-Mental State: A Practical Method For Grading The Cognitive State of Patients for the Clinician', *Journal of Psychiatric Research*, 12, 189–98

Kolanowski, A.M. 1995, 'Disturbing Behaviors in Demented Elders: A Concept Synthesis', *Archives of Psychiatric Nursing*, 9 (4): 188–94.

Logsdon, R.G., Teri, L., Weiner, M.F., Gibbons, L.E., Raskin, M., Peskind, E., Grundman, M., Koss, E., Thomas, R.G. & Thal, L.J. 1999, 'Assessment of Agitation in Alzheimer's Disease: The Agitated Behavior in Dementia Scale', Alzheimer's Disease Cooperative Study, *Journal of the American Geriatrics Society*, 47 (11), 1354–8.

Martino-Saltzman, D., Blasch, B., Morris, R. & McNeal, L. 1991, 'Travel Behavior of Nursing Home Residents Perceived as Wanderers and Non-wanderers', *Gerontologist*, 11, 666–72.

Mattis, S. 1976, 'Mental Status Examination for Organic Mental Syndrome in the Elderly Patient', in L. Bellack & T.B. Karasu (eds), *Geriatric Psychiatry: A Handbook for Psychiatrists and Primary Care Physicians*, pp 77–121, Grune & Stratton, New York.

Monsour, N. & Robb, S. 1982, 'Wandering Behavior in Old Age: A Psychosocial Study', *Social Work*, 27, 411–16.

NANDA: Nursing Diagnosis: Definition & Classification 2001–2002, 4th edn, 1998–2001. Nursecom, Inc.

Reisberg, B., Ferris, S.H., deLeon, M.J. & Crook, T. 1988, 'The Global Deterioration Scale for the Assessment of Primary Degenerative Dementia', *American Journal of Psychiatry*, 139, 1136–9.

Rockwood, K., Stolee, P. & Brahim, A. 1991, 'Outcomes of Admission to a Psychogeriatric Service', *Canadian Journal of Psychiatry*, 36, 275–9.

Sheik, J. & Yesavage, J. 1986, 'Geriatric Depression Scale (GDS): Recent Evidence and Development of a Shorter Version', *Clinical Gerontology*, 37, 819–20.

Siegler, E.L., Capezuti, E., Maislin, G., Baumgarten, M., Evans, L. & Strumpf, N. 1997, 'Effects of a Restraint Reduction Intervention and OBRA '87 Regulations on Psychoactive Drug Use in Nursing Homes', *Journal of the American Geriatrics Society*, 45 (7), 791–6.

Chapter 12 Dysfunctional Behaviour

Ballard, G.B., O'Brien, J., James, I. & Swann, A. 2000, in *Dementia: Management of Behavioural and Psychological Symptoms*, p. 63, Oxford University Press, UK.

Committee on Safety of Medicines 2004, *Atypical antipsychotic drugs and stroke*: message from Professor Gordon Duff, chairman Committee on Safety of Medicines (CEM/CMO/2004/1) <www.mca.gov.uk/ aboutagency/regframework/csm/csmhome.htm> 09/03/04

New Shorter Oxford English Dictionary 1997, Version 1.0.03 (on CD-Rom).

NSOED, see New Shorter Oxford English Dictionary,

Patel, V. & Hope, R.A. 1992, 'A Rating Scale for Aggressive Behaviour in the Elderly—the RAGE', *Psychological Medicine*, 22, 211–21

Royal College of General Practitioners 2004, Guidance for the management of behavioural and psychiatric symptoms in dementia and the treatment of psychosis in people with a history of stroke/ TIA.

SIGN, see Scottish Intercollegiate Guidelines Network (SIGN).

Chapter 13 Pain Management

AHCPR, see Agency for Health Care Policy and Research.

Agency for Health Care Policy and Research 1992, Acute Pain Management Guideline Panel, *Acute Pain Management. Operative or Medical Procedures and Trauma. Clinical Practice Guideline*, AHCPR Pub. No. 92-0032, AHCPR, Public Health Service, US Department of Health and Human Services, Rockville, USA.

AMH, see *Australian Medicines Handbook*.

Australian Medicines Handbook 2002, Finsbury Press, Thebarton, Adelaide.

Butler, R.N. & Gastel, B. 1980, *Care of the Aged: Perspectives on Pain and Discomfort*, in Ng, L.K. & Bonica, J. (eds), *Pain, Discomfort and Humanitarian Care*, pp 297–311, Elsevier North Holland, New York.

Clinch, D., Banerjee, A.K. & Ostic, G. 1984, 'Absence of Abdominal Pain in Elderly Patients with Peptic Ulcer Disease', *Age & Aging*, 13: 120–3

Department of Human Services 1998, 'Therapeutic Guidelines: Analgesics', 1997–1998, 3rd edn, Victoria, Australia.

DHS, see Department of Human Services.

Dryden, J. 2001, 'The Indian Emperor', cited in *Collins Quotation Finder*, HarperCollins.

Hawthorn J. & Redmond, K. (eds) 1998, *Pain Causes and Management*, Blackwell Science, Oxford.

IASP, see International Association for the Study of Pain.

International Association for the Study of Pain 1979, Subcommittee on Taxonomy, 'Pain Terms: A List with Definitions and Notes on Usage', *Pain* (6) 249–52.

Macdonald, J.B. 1984, 'Presentation of Acute Myocardial Infarction in the Elderly', *Age & Aging*, 13: 196–200.

Macintyre, P. & Ready, B.L. 2001, *Acute Pain Management. A Practical Guide*, W B Saunders, London.

Pasero, C., Reed, B.A. & McCaffery, M. 1999, 'Pain in the Elderly', in McCaffery M, & Pasero, C. (eds), *Pain Clinical Manual for Nursing Practice*, p. 675, C.V. Mosby Company, Philadelphia.

WHO 2003, 'WHO Analgesic Ladder', available at various sites, for example, <www.scinfo.org/ PAINN2002/sld029.htm>.

Chapter 14 Palliative Care

Abbey, J. 1998, 'Breaking the Silence: Palliation for People with Dementia', in J. Parker & S. Aranda (eds) 1998, pp 172–86, op. cit.

Alzheimer's Australia 2003, *The Dementia Epidemic: Economic Impact and Positive Solutions for Australia*, Access Economics, Canberra.

ASGM, *see* Australian Society for Geriatric Medicine.

Australian Society for Geriatric Medicine 2001, 'Position Statement No 9: Medical Care for People in Residential Aged Care Services, *Australasian Journal on Ageing*, 20(4), 204–8.

Hudson, R. 1997, 'Documented Life and Death in a Nursing Home', in J. Richmond (ed.), *Nursing Documentation: Writing What We Do*, pp 29–38, Ausmed Publications, Melbourne.

Hudson, R. & Richmond, J. 1998, 'The Meaning of Death in Residential Aged Care', in J. Parker & S. Aranda (eds) 1988, pp 292–302, op. cit.

Hudson, R. & Richmond, J. 2000, *Living, Dying, Caring: Life and Death in a Nursing Home*. Ausmed Publications, Melbourne.

Kellehear, A. 1999, *Health Promoting Palliative Care*, Oxford University Press, Oxford.

Lynn, J. 2001, *Center to Improve the Care of the Dying*, <www. gwu.edu/~cicd>.

MacDonald, A., Carpenter, I.G., Box, O., Roberts, A. & Sahu, S. 2002, Dementia and use of psychotropic medication in non 'Elderly Mentally Infirm' nursing homes in South East England. *Age and Ageing*, 31: 58–64.

Parker, J. & Aranda, S. (eds) 1988, *Palliative Care: Explorations and Challenges*, Maclennan & Petty, Sydney.

Saunders, C. & Baines, M. 1989, *Living with Dying: The Management of Terminal Disease*, 2nd edn, OUP, Oxford.

Chapter 15 Care Plans

Orlando, I.J. 1961, *The Dynamic Nurse–Patient Relationship, Function, Process and Principles*, G.P. Putnam, New York.

Orlando, I.J. 1972, *The Discipline and Teaching of Nursing Process: An Evaluative Study*, New G.P. Putnam, New York.

Chapter 16 Delirium and Dementia

Breitbart, W., Gibson, C. & Tremblay, A. 2002, 'The Delirium Experience: Delirium Recall and Delirium-related Distress in Hospitalised Patients', *Psychomatics* 43:3; 183–91.

Cole, M.G., Primeau, F.J. & Elie, L.M. 1990, 'Delirium: Prevention, Treatment and Outcome Studies', *Journal of Geriatric Psychiatry and Neurology*, 11: 126–37.

Cummings, J.L. 1986, 'Subcortical Dementia: Neuropsychology, Neuropsychiatry and Pathophysiology', *BJP*, 149: 682–97.

Edlund, A., Lundstrom, M., Brannstrom, B., Bucht, G. & Gustafonson, Y. 2001, 'Delirium before and after Operation for Femoral Neck Fracture', *Journal of the American Geriatric Society*, 49: 1335–40.

Fick, D., Agostini, J. & Inouye, S. 2002, 'Delirium Superimposed on Dementia: A Systemic Review', *American Geriatric Society*, 50: 1723–32.

Folstein, M.F., Folstein, S.E. & McHugh, P.R. 1975, 'Mini-Mental State: A Practical Method For Grading The Cognitive State of Patients for the Clinician', *Journal of Psychiatric Research*, 12, 189–98.

Hall, K. & Hassett, A. 1998, 'Assessing and Managing Old Age Psychiatric Disorders in Community Practice', *Medical Journal of Australia*, <www.mja.com.au>.

Inouye, S.K. & Charpentier, P.A. 1996, 'Precipitating Factors for Delirium in Hospitalised Older People', JAMA, 275: 852–7.

Inouye, S.K. 1998, 'Delirium in Hospitalised Older Patients: Recognition and Risk Factors', *Journal of Geriatric Psychiatry & Neurology*, 11: 118–24.

MacDonald, A. et al. 2002 ibid.

McLean, S. 1987, 'Assessing Dementia: Difficulties, Definitions and Differential Diagnosis', *Australian and New Zealand Journal of Psychiatry*, 21: 142–74.

McLean, S. 1993, 'Practical Management of Alzheimers Disease', *Modern Medicine of Australia*, 4: 16–27.

Meagher, D.J. 2001, 'Delirium: the Role of Psychiatry', *Advances in Psychiatric Treatment*, 7: 433–42.

O'Keefe, S. 1999, 'Delirium in the Elderly', *Age & Aging*, 28: 5–8.

Chapter 17 Medications

Cunningham, G., Dodd, T.R.P., Grant, D.J., McMurdo, M & Richards, R.M.E. 1997, Drug-related problems in elderly patients admitted to Tayside hospitals, methods for prevention and subsequent reassessment. *Age and Ageing*, 26, 375–82.

Mannesse, C.K., Derkx, F.H., deRidder, M.A., van der Cammen, T.J. & Man in't Veld, A.J. 1997, Adverse drug reactions in elderly patients as contributing factor for hospital admissions: cross-sectional study. *BMJ*, 315, 1057–8.

Mannesse, C.K., Derkx, F.H., deRidder, M.A., Man in't Veld, A.J & van der Cammen, T.J. 2000, Contribution of adverse drug reactions to hospital admission of older patients. *Age and Ageing*, 29, 35–9.

Shock, N.W. 1962, 'The Physiology of Aging', *Scientific American*, 1(168): 100–8.

WHO, *see* World Health Organization.

World Health Organization 1981, 'Health Care in the Elderly: Report of the Technical Group on the Use of Medications in the Elderly', *Drugs*, 22: 279.

Chapter 18 Complementary Therapies

Hudson R (ed) 2003, *Dementia Nursing: A Guide to Practice*, Ausmed Publications, Melbourne.

NHACT, *see Nurse's Handbook of Alternative & Complementary Therapies*.

Nurse's Handbook of Alternative & Complementary Therapies 1999, Springhouse Corporation, Pennsylvania, USA.

Chapter 19 Cultural Differences

Dartington, T. 1980, *Family Care of Old People*, Souvenir Press, London.

Fineman, N. 1991, 'The Social Construction of Noncompliance: Implications for Cross-Cultural Geriatric Practice', *Journal of Cross-Cultural Gerontology*, 6, 219–28.

Chapter 20 Occupational Health and Safety

Health and Safety at Work, Act 1974, *HMSO*, London.

WH&S *see* Workplace Health & Safety.

Workplace Health & Safety 1989, 'Audit Program, Division of Workplace Health & Safety', AP 002, Department of Employment, Vocational Education, Training and Industrial Relations (Queensland).

Chapter 21 Elder Abuse

Baker, A.A. 1975, 'Granny Bashing', *Modern Geriatrics*, 5: 20–4.

Callahan, J.J. 1988, 'Elder Abuse: Some Questions for Policy Makers', *The Gerontologist*, 28: 453–8.

Council of Europe 1992, *Violence Against Elderly People*, Council of Europe Press, Strasbourg.

Davies, M. 1994, 'Recognising Abuse: An Assessment Tool for Nurses', in P. Decalmer & F. Glendenning (eds), *The Mistreatment of Elderly People*, pp 102–16, Sage Publications, London.

Dolon, R. & Hendricks, J.E. 1989, 'An Exploratory Study Comparing Attitudes and Practices of Police Officers and Social Service Providers in Elder Abuse and Neglect Cases', *Journal of Elder Abuse and Neglect*, 1(1): 75–90.

Eckley, S.C.A. &Vilakazi, P.A.C. 1995, 'Elder Abuse in South Africa', in J.I. Kosberg & J.L. Garcia (eds), *Elder Abuse: International and Cross-Cultural Perspectives*, pp 171–82, The Haworth Press, Inc., New York.

Fleishman, R. & Ronen, R. 1989, 'Quality of Care and Maltreatment in Israel's Institutions for the Elderly', in R.S. Wolf & S. Bergman (eds), *Stress, Conflict and Abuse of the Elderly*, JDC-Brookdale Institute of Gerontology, Jerusalem.

Giordano, N.H. & Giordano, J.A. 1984, 'Elder Abuse: A Review of the Literature', *Social Work*, 29(2): 232–6.

Hudson, M.F. & Johnson, T.F. 1987, 'Elder Neglect and Abuse: A Review of the Literature', in M.C. Eisdorfer (ed.), *Annual Review of Gerontology*, Springer, New York.

Hugman, R. 1995, 'The Implications of the Term 'Elder Abuse' for Problem Definition in Health and Social Welfare', *Journal of Social Policy*, 24: 493–507.

Hugman, R. 2000, 'The Value of Old Age in Modern Society: Social Responses to "Elder Abuse"', in W.T. Liu & H. Kendig (eds), *Who Should Care for the Elderly? An East–West Value Divide*, pp 143–61, Singapore University Press, Singapore.

Jones, G. 1992, 'A Communication Model for Dementia', in G. Jones and B.M.L. Mieson (eds), *Caregiving in Dementia: Research and Applications*, Routledge, London.

Kent Social Services Department 1989, *Practice Guidelines for Dealing with Elder Abuse*, Policy Officer, Kent County Council, Canterbury (UK).

Kosberg, J.I. 1988, 'Preventing elder abuse', *The Gerontologist*, 28: 43–50.

Kurrle, S.E., Sadler, P.M. & Cameron, I.D. 1991, 'Elder abuse—An Australian Case Series', *Medical Journal of Australia*, 155: 150–3.

Leroux, T.G. & Petrunik, M. 1990, 'The Construction of Elder Abuse as a Social Problem: A Canadian Perspective', *International Journal of Health Services*, 20: 651–63.

Manthorpe, J. 1994, 'Elder Abuse and Key Areas in Social Work', in P. Decalmer & F. Glendenning (eds), *The Mistreatment of Elderly People*, pp 88–101, Sage Publications, London.

Ministry of Citizenship 1991, *A Review of Community/Program Responses to Elder Abuse in Ontario*, Canada Printing, Ontario.

Moore, T. & Thompson, T. 1987, 'Elder Abuse: A Review of Research, Programmes and Policy', *Social Worker*, 55(3): 115–22.

Schlesinger, B. & Schlesinger, R. (eds) 1988, *Abuse of the Elderly, Issues and Annotated Bibliography*, University of Toronto Press, Toronto.

Slevin, O. 1991, 'Ageist Attitudes among Young Adults: Implications for a Caring Profession', *Journal of Advanced Nursing*, 16: 1197–205.

Sumner, K. 2002, No Secrets. The Protection of Vulnerable Adults from Abuse: local codes of practice. Centre for Policy on Ageing, London.

Chapter 22 Communicating in Frustrating Situations

Beck, C., Ortigara, A., Mercer, S. & Shue, V. 1999, 'Enabling and Empowering Certified Nursing Assistants for Quality Dementia Care', *International Journal of Geriatric Psychiatry*, 14: 197–212.

Done, D. & Thomas, J. 2001, 'Training in Communication Skills for Informal Carers of People Suffering from Dementia: A Cluster Randomized Clinical Trial Comparing a Therapist-led Workshop and Booklet', *International Journal of Geriatric Psychiatry*, 16: 816–21.

Eliopoulos, C. 1987, *Gerontological Nursing*, 2nd edn, J.B. Lippincott Company, Philadelphia, USA.

Feil, N. 1993, *The Validation Breakthrough*, Health Professions Press Inc. Baltimore.

Finnema, E., Droes, R., Ribbe, M. & Van Tilburg, W. 2000, 'The Effects of Emotion-Orientated Approaches to Care for Persons Suffering from Dementia: A Review of the Literature', *International Journal of Geriatric Psychiatry*, 15: 141–61.

Forster, S. 2003, 'Reminiscence', in Hudson R. (ed.) 2003, *Dementia Nursing A Guide to Practice*, pp 283–4, Ausmed Publications, Melbourne, Victoria.

Meier, S. 2002, *Communication Series-Communication Styles*, Strategic Search Consultants-Online.com.

Pinkney M. & Whiter B. (eds) 1997, *Pocket Positives*, The Five Mile Press, Noble Park, Australia.

Queensland Health 1998, *Cultural Diversity: A Guide for Health Professionals*, Queensland Government, Australia.

Ward, R. 2002, 'Dementia, Communication, and Care: 1. Expanding Our Understanding', *The Journal of Dementia Care*, Sept/Oct: 33–5.

Ward, R. 2002, 'Dementia, Communication and Care: 2. Communication in Context', *The Journal of Dementia Care*, Nov/Dec 33–7.

Index